NUTRITION AND DIET RESEARCH PROGRESS

FOOD PRODUCTS USE OF VOLUNTARY HEALTH- AND NUTRITION-RELATED CLAIMS

NUTRITION AND DIET RESEARCH PROGRESS

Additional books in this series can be found on Nova's website under the Series tab.

Additional E-books in this series can be found on Nova's website under the E-book tab.

PUBLIC HEALTH IN THE 21ST CENTURY

Additional books in this series can be found on Nova's website under the Series tab.

Additional E-books in this series can be found on Nova's website under the E-book tab.

NUTRITION AND DIET RESEARCH PROGRESS

FOOD PRODUCTS USE OF VOLUNTARY HEALTH- AND NUTRITION-RELATED CLAIMS

OREN CHERTOK
AND
MARCUS ABERLIEB
EDITORS

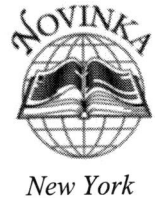

New York

Copyright © 2013 by Nova Science Publishers, Inc.

All rights reserved. No part of this book may be reproduced, stored in a retrieval system or transmitted in any form or by any means: electronic, electrostatic, magnetic, tape, mechanical photocopying, recording or otherwise without the written permission of the Publisher.

For permission to use material from this book please contact us:
Telephone 631-231-7269; Fax 631-231-8175
Web Site: http://www.novapublishers.com

NOTICE TO THE READER

The Publisher has taken reasonable care in the preparation of this book, but makes no expressed or implied warranty of any kind and assumes no responsibility for any errors or omissions. No liability is assumed for incidental or consequential damages in connection with or arising out of information contained in this book. The Publisher shall not be liable for any special, consequential, or exemplary damages resulting, in whole or in part, from the readers' use of, or reliance upon, this material. Any parts of this book based on government reports are so indicated and copyright is claimed for those parts to the extent applicable to compilations of such works.

Independent verification should be sought for any data, advice or recommendations contained in this book. In addition, no responsibility is assumed by the publisher for any injury and/or damage to persons or property arising from any methods, products, instructions, ideas or otherwise contained in this publication.

This publication is designed to provide accurate and authoritative information with regard to the subject matter covered herein. It is sold with the clear understanding that the Publisher is not engaged in rendering legal or any other professional services. If legal or any other expert assistance is required, the services of a competent person should be sought. FROM A DECLARATION OF PARTICIPANTS JOINTLY ADOPTED BY A COMMITTEE OF THE AMERICAN BAR ASSOCIATION AND A COMMITTEE OF PUBLISHERS.

Additional color graphics may be available in the e-book version of this book.

Library of Congress Cataloging-in-Publication Data

ISBN: 978-1-62808-440-5

Published by Nova Science Publishers, Inc. † New York

CONTENTS

Preface		vii
Chapter 1	Introduction of New Food Products with Voluntary Health- and Nutrition-Related Claims, 1989-2010 *Steve W. Martinez*	**1**
Chapter 2	Do Food Labels Make a Difference? ... Sometimes *Elise Golan, Fred Kuchler and Barry Krissoff*	**63**
Index		**73**

PREFACE

Voluntary health- and nutrition-related claims by food companies were present on 43.1 percent of new products introduced in 2010. Health- and nutrition-related claims such as "low fat," "low cholesterol," or "high fiber" potentially influence consumer purchases and can lead companies to reformulate their less healthy products to qualify for the claims; hence, it is important to understand food companies' adoption of these claims. This book tracks health- and nutrition-related claims on new U.S. food and beverage products from 1989 to 2010 and delineates the claims by product category and type of claim. Over the 2009 to 2010 period, the sales and average nutrient content of all new food and beverage products carrying at least one of the top ten health- and nutrition-related claims is also analyzed.

Chapter 1 - This study tracks food products introduced from 1989 to 2010 to better understand the adoption of voluntary health- and nutrition-related claims by companies. New food products introduced with health- and nutrition-related claims accounted for 43.1 percent of all new U.S. food product introductions in 2010, up from 25.2 percent in 2001 and 34.6 percent in 1989. The reduction in health- and nutrition-related claims from 1989 to 2001 followed enactment of the Nutrition Labeling and Education Act of 1990 (NLEA). The NLEA required most food products to carry the Nutrition Facts label and established labeling rules for the use of voluntary nutrient content and health claims. Overall growth in health- and nutrition-related claims after 2001 reflect increases in low/no calorie, whole grain, high fiber, and low/no sugar claims, along with relatively new claims related to no gluten, no trans fats, antioxidants, and omega-3. This period was characterized by nutrition information and education campaigns targeting obesity. Recent increases in health- and nutrition-related claim use also reflect evolving consumer needs and preferences for foods that promote a healthy lifestyle and disease-fighting capabilities, and new labeling regulations directed at trans fats.

Chapter 2 –

- Competition drives food manufacturers to voluntarily label their products' desirable attributes and to use third-party certifiers to bolster credibility.
- Mandatory food labeling is usually more successful at filling information gaps than at addressing externalities such as environmental or health spillovers associated with food production and consumption
- Mandatory labeling may initially have a larger impact on manufacturers' production decisions than on consumers' food choices.

There is a lot to know about the food we eat. The ingredients in a jar of spaghetti sauce, a box of cereal, or a cup of coffee could come from around the corner or around the world; they could be processed by children or by high-tech machines; they could be grown on huge corporate farms or on small family-run farms; or they could be mostly artificial or 100-percent natural.

While a description of a food product could include information on a multitude of attributes, not all of them are important to consumers or regulators. Information on some attributes could affect the health and welfare of consumers by influencing their food choices. Information on other attributes might have no effect at all.

Consumers, food companies, third-party entities, and governments play a role in determining which attributes are described on the label. The interaction of these groups influences which information is labeled voluntarily, which is mandated, and which is not labeled at all. It shapes the way information is presented and the accuracy and credibility of that information. The economics behind food labeling provides insight into the dynamics of voluntary food labeling and the types of market failures best addressed through mandatory labeling requirements.

In: Food Products Use ...
Editors: O. Chertok and M. Aberlieb

ISBN: 978-1-62808-440-5
© 2013 Nova Science Publishers, Inc.

Chapter 1

INTRODUCTION OF NEW FOOD PRODUCTS WITH VOLUNTARY HEALTH- AND NUTRITION-RELATED CLAIMS, 1989-2010[*]

Steve W. Martinez

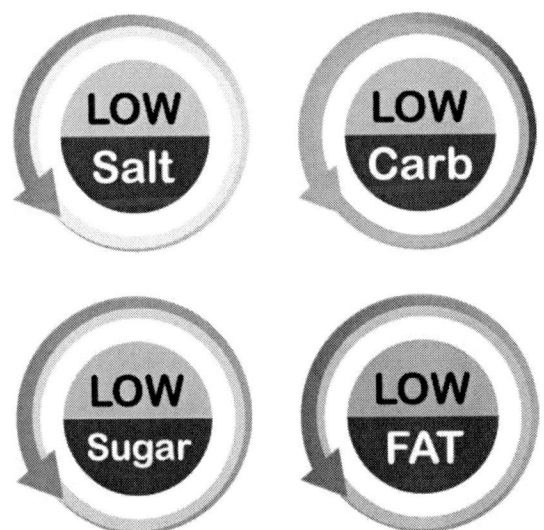

Photo: Shutterstock.

---

[*] This is an edited, reformatted and augmented version of United States Department of Agriculture, Economic Research Service, Economic Information Bulletin Number 108, dated February 2013.

Abstract

This study tracks food products introduced from 1989 to 2010 to better understand the adoption of voluntary health- and nutrition-related claims by companies. New food products introduced with health- and nutrition-related claims accounted for 43.1 percent of all new U.S. food product introductions in 2010, up from 25.2 percent in 2001 and 34.6 percent in 1989. The reduction in health- and nutrition-related claims from 1989 to 2001 followed enactment of the Nutrition Labeling and Education Act of 1990 (NLEA). The NLEA required most food products to carry the Nutrition Facts label and established labeling rules for the use of voluntary nutrient content and health claims. Overall growth in health- and nutrition-related claims after 2001 reflect increases in low/no calorie, whole grain, high fiber, and low/no sugar claims, along with relatively new claims related to no gluten, no trans fats, antioxidants, and omega-3. This period was characterized by nutrition information and education campaigns targeting obesity. Recent increases in health- and nutrition-related claim use also reflect evolving consumer needs and preferences for foods that promote a healthy lifestyle and disease-fighting capabilities, and new labeling regulations directed at trans fats.

Summary

What Is the Issue?

Voluntary health- and nutrition-related claims by food companies were present on 43.1 percent of new products introduced in 2010. Health- and nutrition-related claims such as "low fat," "low cholesterol," or "high fiber" potentially influence consumer purchases and can lead companies to reformulate their less healthy products to qualify for the claims; hence, it is important to understand food companies' adoption of these claims.

This study tracks health- and nutrition-related claims on new U.S. food and beverage products from 1989 to 2010 and delineates the claims by product category and type of claim. Over the 2009 to 2010 period, we also evaluate sales and average nutrient content of all new food and beverage products carrying at least 1 of the top 10 health- and nutrition-related claims from 2010.

What Did the Study Find?

The percentage of food products making health- and nutrition-related claims fell between 1989 and 2001, while the number of claims per product increased. The overall percentage decrease in claims followed the Nutrition Labeling and Education Act (NLEA) of 1990, which was implemented in 1993/1994. The act made the Nutrition Facts label mandatory and established rules for the use of voluntary health- and nutrition-related claims on food and beverage products, such as those related to low/no fat, low/no cholesterol, and high fiber. This suggests that the NLEA may have led to reductions in overall claim usage by preventing non-qualifying products from using specific claims. In addition, the number of claims per product increased from 2.0 in 1989 to 2.2 in 2001. This suggests that the NLEA did not undermine the competitive process, but may have contributed to its expansion by establishing a credible means of disclosing health and nutritional characteristics.

From 2001 to 2010, health- and nutrition-related claims became an increasingly important feature of new product introductions. Health- and nutrition-related claims per product continued to increase, from 2.2 in 2001 to 2.6 in 2010, which suggests that competition between companies continued to result in a more complete representation of the health and nutritional attributes of their products. A proliferation of new products with claims appealing to weight-conscious consumers over 2001 to 2010 reflects growing awareness of obesity-related problems and educational campaigns targeting obesity. Claims related to gluten, antioxidants, and omega-3 ranked among the leading health- and nutrition-related claims by 2010. Growing consumer demand for food products that contribute to overall health beyond basic nutrition may have provided manufacturers with incentives to supply and promote these products. The largest increase in health- and nutrition-related claims over 2001 to 2010 was for "no gluten," followed by "no trans fats." The growth in "no trans fats" claims came as companies responded to new food labeling regulations that required disclosure of the trans fats content, and public communications that gave prominence to limiting trans fatty acids. For new food products introduced in 2009 and 2010, sales and nutritional quality of those products carrying health- and nutrition-related claims exceeded that of all new food products.

How Was the Study Conducted?

This report relies primarily on data from the Product Launch Analytics database, developed by the Datamonitor Group. We used the database to track new products carrying health- and nutrition-related claims from 1989 to 2010. Datamonitor's field research team collected information across 20 elements for each new product in the database, including brand, product category (e.g., snacks, cereal, and dairy), package size, ingredients, and most common marketing messages or claims made on packages. The team also provided a qualitative product description. We used Mintel's Global New Product Database (Mintel GNPD) to compare the nutritional profile of new products with health- and nutrition-related claims to all new products over 2009 to 2010. We used data provided through a partnership between Mintel and Symphony IRI (formerly Information Resources, Inc., or IRI) to compare sales of new products in Mintel GNPD over the same period.

INTRODUCTION

One way that food companies can influence consumer purchases is through the use of voluntary health- and nutrition-related (HNR) claims (e.g., "low fat," "high fiber"). They provide a means for companies to differentiate their products by identifying foods that are high or low in specific nutrients, which may assist consumers in improving the nutritional quality of their diet. Sales of products with fat-, sodium-, and calorie-related claims accounted for $73 billion in 2009 (*Nielsenwire*, 2010) or 12 percent of food sales for at-home consumption.[1] Past studies of HNR claims have mostly focused on impacts on product evaluations and purchase decisions of consumers, as opposed to understanding the adoption of HNR claims by companies (Roe, Levy, and Derby, 1999; Van Camp et al., 2010). Studies of companies' adoption of HNR claims over periods of changing claims regulation, new health and nutrition information, and changing consumer preferences complement studies of claim effects on consumers' product evaluations and purchase intentions.

This study tracks food product introductions carrying HNR claims from 1989 to 2010. New product introductions were delineated along several dimensions including types of HNR claims used, their frequency, and types of products making claims. By tracing new product introductions over an extended period of time, we can document changes in product claims by companies as: food labeling regulations are changed, new health and nutrition information is identified, and consumer needs and preferences change. Unlike previous studies of HNR claims on new products, this study also tracks sales of all products introduced in 2009 and 2010 to compare purchase patterns of products with health- and nutrient-related claims to all new products. New products with HNR claims will have little impact on diet and health unless they are purchased by consumers. Over the same period, we also compare the average nutritional profile of products with HNR claims to all new products to assess whether the claims could assist consumers in choosing more nutritious products. This study also addresses recommendations from the White House Task Force on Childhood Obesity Report to the President (2010), which include encouraging industries to shift product portfolios to promote new and reformulated foods and beverages that are healthier. Previous progress in this area is analyzed by tracking the introduction of products that assist consumers in identifying "healthier" formulations, such as low fat, low or no sodium, and less or no sugar. Sales of these products are also evaluated to determine whether they may account for an increasing share of consumer purchases of new products. Unless otherwise noted, we define "new" to include seven types of product introductions, following the nomenclature used by the Datamonitor Group, a business information and market analysis company:

1. New flavor(s) of an existing product line.
2. New package size.
3. New packaging formats (for example, a brand of mayonnaise formerly available only in glass jars is introduced in plastic squeeze bottles.)
4. Newly available within the country.
5. Significantly reformulated (for example, a drink mix is reformulated to contain 47 percent less sugar.)
6. Renamed.
7. An entirely new product or product line.

INCENTIVES TO MARKET NEW FOOD PRODUCTS USING VOLUNTARY HEALTH- AND NUTRITION- RELATED CLAIMS

The introduction of a product represents the first stage of the product life cycle, which includes the product's introduction, its growth in market share, maturity, and potential decline in market share (Tanner and Raymond, 2010). All products do not pass through all stages, and the length of a stage may vary. For example, some products may never experience growth and are withdrawn from the market. Estimates of market success rates of new food products vary depending on how "success" is defined. Based on a 1997 analysis by Prime Consulting Group Inc., 33 percent of new products were deemed successful (i.e., those with sales that remained above second quarter sales over a 2-year tracking period), 42 percent were still in distribution but declining in sales, and 25 percent failed by year 2 (*Progressive Grocer*, 1997). Using a different definition of success, IRI analyzed over 600 products introduced between 1996 and 1998 and found that the success rate of new products was 48 percent (Sachdev, 2001). A product was deemed successful if it was distributed in at least 50 percent of national outlets in its first year and didn't lose more than 30 percent of distribution in year 2.

Companies that introduce new products may choose to promote the nutrient and health benefits of their products. New products may be developed and introduced for many reasons, some of which include (IOM, 2010):

- Satisfying changing consumer preferences for healthier products by improving nutritional characteristics, for example, by removing undesirable ingredients;
- Responding to new technologies that make it feasible to create new and reformulated products, such as the development of healthier substitute ingredients (Unnevehr and Jagmanaite, 2008);
- Responding to changes in Government regulations and policies that provide incentives to reformulate products or develop new ones (for example, mandatory disclosure of nutrient content that influences consumer choice of food products (Unnevehr and Jagmanaite, 2008) and lifting of regulatory bans on advertising the health benefits of food products (Ippolito and Mathios, 1990)); and
- Responding to new or improved products introduced by competitors, for example, to compete on nutritional quality as a means of differentiating their products.

Food companies may also introduce reformulated products to avoid public litigation or improve their image. For example, in 2003, a suit against Kraft Foods was filed by a public interest group directed at the health impact of trans fats in its snack foods (Unnevehr and Jagmanaite, 2008). Kraft settled out of court by agreeing to reduce the trans fats content in its popular brands. In addition, companies may attempt to gain a competitive advantage by voluntarily reporting on activities that address responsible social and environmental practices. In 2011, 83 percent of the 100 top U.S. companies reported on corporate responsibility activities through dedicated corporate responsibility or sustainability reports, company websites, or annual financial reports, up from 74 percent in 2008 (KPMG International Cooperative, 2011). Several leading food companies use the Global Reporting Initiative (GRI) index, which provides standardized guidelines for reporting progress on corporate economic, environmental, labor, human rights, social (altruistic), and product responsibility practices. For example, Pepsico, Kellogg Company, and ConAgra Foods describe progress made in lowering fats, added sugars, sodium, and trans fats in the product responsibility component of the index. Enhanced reputation from corporate responsibility reporting to consumers and investors may create incentives for positive corporate behavior (Yach et al., 2010; KPMG International Cooperative, 2011).

Food Labeling Legislation Strictly Regulates Health- and Nutrition-Related Claims

Over the period covered in this study, the most significant piece of food labeling legislation in recent history was passed (Ghani and Childs, 1999). The Nutrition Labeling and Education Act of 1990 (NLEA) established labeling regulations that require most products to carry the Nutrition Facts label. The regulations also include labeling rules for voluntary claims that identify which HNR claims are allowed and under what circumstances they can be used. The proposed regulations were published in 1991, and final rules were released in January 1993 (Ippolito and Mathios, 1993). The regulations, which took effect in May 1994 for nutrient content claims and in May 1993 for health claims, are interpreted and implemented by the Food and Drug Administration (FDA) (Ippolito and Pappalardo, 2002) (see box, "Provisions of the Nutrition Labeling and Education Act of 1990").[2]

The objectives of the NLEA were to reduce consumer confusion about food labels and aid consumers in making healthy food choices. The act was intended to increase the reliability of HNR claims on labels by making it more difficult for food companies to make unsubstantiated claims. By giving manufacturers an opportunity to make positive claims about their products, the NLEA aimed to provide an incentive to increase the availability of more healthful food choices (Brecher et al., 2000).

FDA categorizes HNR claims into nutrient content claims, health claims, qualified health claims, and structure/function claims (U.S. Department of Health and Human Services, 2009):

- *Nutrient content claims* characterize the level of a nutrient found in food, such as "low fat" and "contains 100 calories." Implied nutrient content claims suggest a nutrient is available in a certain amount (e.g., "high in oat bran").
- *Health claims* characterize the presence or absence of a nutrient that is linked to a disease or health-related condition (e.g., "diets low in sodium may reduce the risk of high blood pressure, a disease associated with many factors"). Implied health claims suggest that a relationship exists between the presence or level of a substance in the food and a disease or health-related condition (e.g., vignettes used with specific nutrient information).

Provisions of the Nutrition Labeling and Education Act of 1990 (NLEA)

The NLEA set up a premarket approval requirement for nutrient content and health claims and required the Food and Drug Administration (FDA) to define certain commonly used terms such as "lite" and "healthy" (Silverglade and Heller, 2010). For example, FDA made provisions for how much sodium a product could contain so that claims such as "sodium free," "low sodium," and "reduced sodium" could be used. Prior to the regulations, nutrition and health claims were used by manufacturers without any standardized definition. If a company is interested in establishing a new nutrient content or health claim, it can petition FDA.

Claims are limited to an approved list of nutrients. Most nutrient content claim regulations apply only to nutrients that have an established daily value. For nutrients without an established daily value, a manufacturer may make a claim that specifies the amount of the nutrient per serving (e.g., "X grams of omega-3 fatty acids"), but cannot implicitly characterize the level of the nutrient (U.S. Department of Health and Human Services, 2009).

The new regulations allowed for the use of 11 core terms on food labels: low, free, lean, extra lean, high, more, good source, reduced, less, light, and fewer. Claims that did not conform to the new requirements had to be dropped.

For example, the "X percent fat free" claim could no longer be used unless the product qualified as low fat. In addition, important cross-compliance requirements were established for use of nutrient content claims. If companies make nutrient content claims on their labels, they are required to disclose undesirable characteristics. For example, a product with a "high fiber" claim must have the disclaimer "not a low-fat product" if it does not qualify as low fat.

The NLEA rules also allowed for a limited number of health claims and restricted which foods could make such claims (Ippolito and Mathios, 1993). Foods with excessive levels, as established by FDA, of total fat, saturated fat, cholesterol, or sodium could not carry any health claim on their label. In addition, food must contain at least 10 percent of the recommended daily intake (RDI) or daily reference value (DRY) for vitamin A, vitamin C, iron, calcium, protein, or fiber to qualify for a health claim. There are also regulations specific to a particular health claim that, for example, require the food to meet the definition of "low" or "high" for the nutrient associated with the claim. For example, to qualify for the health claim "diets low in sodium are associated with a low prevalence of hypertension or high blood pressure," a product must meet the criteria for the "low sodium" nutrient content claim.

The NLEA does not cover foods regulated by USDA, which are primarily meat and poultry products (IOM, 2010). USDA voluntarily put in place nutrition labeling regulations consistent with those adopted by FDA. In 1993, USDA made the nutrition labeling of meat and poultry products mandatory, except for single-ingredient, raw products (IOM, 2010). In addition, it made similar provisions to that of FDA regarding nutritional claims. Beginning on March 1, 2012, nutrition-information labeling requirements became mandatory for single-ingredient, raw products and ground or chopped meat and poultry.

The NLEA also does not apply to advertisements, such as those in magazines and on websites, which are under the authority of the Federal Trade Commission (FTC). In May 1994, the FTC issued a policy statement harmonizing advertising policy with the new food labeling rules (Ippolito and Pappalardo, 2002). All advertising claims are subject to general advertising enforcement under the FTC's authority to pursue deceptive business practices. While advertisers are not directly bound by the FDA rules, FTC policy guidance states that claims not in compliance with the FDA rules will receive careful scrutiny from the FTC.

- *Qualified health claims* differ from health claims in that they must be accompanied by a disclaimer (e.g., "scientific evidence suggests but does not prove that eating 1.5 ounces per day of most nuts [such as name of specific nut] as part of a diet low in saturated fat and cholesterol may reduce the risk of heart disease").
- *Structure/function claims* describe how a product affects the structure or function of the body, but do not imply a relationship to a disease (e.g., "calcium builds strong bones").

Previous studies suggest that most HNR claims are nutrient content claims, followed by structure/function claims and health claims. For example, based on FDA's 2000-2001 Food Label and Package Survey (FLAPS), 49.7 percent of packaged foods sold at supermarkets were estimated to have a nutrient content claim, compared to 6.2 percent with a structure/function claim and 4.4 percent with a health claim (LeGault et al., 2004).[3]

Three possible responses by manufacturers to the new regulations were identified by Caswell et al. (2003).

First, companies that did not previously use claims on products that met the standards for claims could have begun using them under the new regulations.

Second, companies making claims may have dropped them because the claims did not meet the newly detailed requirements.

Third, because access to information on nutrition quality is improved, manufacturers may reformulate their less nutritious products to qualify for HNR claims to differentiate their products from the competition. Overall, the number of HNR claims following the new regulations could have risen or fallen, depending on these possible manufacturing responses.

Studies have noted other possible reasons for reductions in the use of HNR claims following the NLEA. Claim usage may fall if disclosure requirements made them more costly to implement or reduced their effectiveness, since companies that make nutrient claims must also highlight undesirable attributes (Ippolito and Pappalardo, 2002; Ippolito and Mathios, 1993). Padberg (1992) raised the possibility that manufacturers would not use standardized claims because products would appear alike, and therefore they would compete based on non-nutritional criteria, such as taste and packaging.

Do Health- and Nutrition-Related Claims Affect the Purchase Decision?

Some researchers have argued that using HNR claims to advertise new products serves a different and effective function in communicating nutritional information to a broader range of consumers than the Nutrition Facts label alone (Caswell et al., 2003). Kozup et al. (2003), for instance, concluded that presenting consumers with favorable nutrition information or health claims leads to positive effects on attitudes toward the product and purchase intentions, and reduces the perceived disease risk. In addition, information from the Nutrition Facts label does not moderate the effects of a health claim. Ford et al. (1996) concluded that health claims and nutrition information have independent effects on perceptions of product healthfulness when both types of information are presented. Kim et al. (2001) compared the impact of the Nutrition Facts label, serving sizes, nutrient content claims, list of ingredients, and health claims on diet quality. They found that, while all lead to healthier diets, consumers' use of health claims has the greatest impact. Levy et al. (1999) concluded that nutrient and health claims influence consumer perceptions of the healthfulness of products and positively affect purchase behavior for specific product categories and claims. Harris et al. (2011) found that nutrition-related claims on children's cereals made parents more likely to buy the cereals. Reported declines in the use of the Nutrition Facts label could be due to information costs associated with comparing products using the Nutrition Facts label and consumers' preference for abbreviated health and front label claims (Kiesel and Villas-Boas, 2010; Carlson, 2010).

Ippolito and Mathios (1991) concluded that producer advertising of the health benefits of their products may have positive impacts on the consumption of healthier products beyond that of government and other sources of health information. This is because producers bring additional resources to advertise health benefits, and they are more likely to use advertising media and methods that reach a broader population.

Several studies have examined the effects of HNR claims in experimental settings. In the presence of a Nutrition Facts label, health and nutrition claims on the front of a package were found not to have a positive effect on consumers' evaluation of product healthfulness (Garretson and Burton, 2000; Teratanavat et al., 2004; Keller et al., 1997; Mitra et al., 1999) or purchase intentions (Garretson and Burton, 2000; Keller et al., 1997). In addition, inconsistencies between a claim and information from the Nutrition Facts label can reduce trust in the manufacturer and the claim (Garretson and Burton,

2000; Keller et al., 1997). On the other hand, Wansink and Chandon (2006) concluded that "low fat" nutrition claims lead overweight consumers to overeat snack foods by increasing serving sizes and reducing consumption guilt.

Others have found more complex relationships between how consumers use Nutrition Facts labels and voluntary health- and nutrition-related claims. For example, Drewnowski et al. (2010) found that consumer perception of product healthfulness was most strongly driven by proclaimed presence of protein, fiber, vitamin C, and calcium, and absence of saturated fat and sodium, but less influenced by sugar, total fat, and vitamin A content claims. In addition, nutrient content claims had a much greater influence on women compared to men. Kemp et al. (2007) found that consumers who are more motivated to process nutrition information are also more likely to use information from the Nutrition Facts label, less likely to purchase a product based only on nutrient claims, and better able to link certain nutrition information to disease risk perceptions. The effect of HNR claims on purchases is further complicated by the importance of taste compared to nutritional quality when making purchase decisions (Drichoutis et al., 2006; Chandon and Wansink, 2011; Stewart, Blisard, and Jolliffe, 2006; Moorman et al., 2012; Glanz et al., 1998; French et al., 1999).

Consumers' use of HNR claims may also be affected by information linking diet and health, which may increase consumer demand for healthier product formulations. Public nutrition education efforts, such as those that implement the Federal *Dietary Guidelines for Americans*, may influence public awareness and understanding of diet and health linkages (Dharmasena et al., 2011). Szykman et al. (1997) concluded that programs designed to educate consumers about the effectiveness of diet in combating and preventing disease may lead to greater use of package claims and nutrition labels. Changes in consumer interest in the nutrition attributes of products is expected to affect food companies' voluntary use of marketing claims of superiority with respect to one or more nutrients (Caswell et al., 2003).

DATAMONITOR TRACKS NEW FOOD AND BEVERAGE PRODUCT INTRODUCTIONS

This report relies extensively on Datamonitor's Product Launch Analytics (PLA) database, which provides updated information on new product introductions 24 hours a day, 5 days per week. A field research team collects information across 20 elements for each product in the database, including brand, product category (e.g., snacks, cereal, dairy), package size, ingredients, and most common marketing messages or claims made on packages. A qualitative product description is also provided. For a product to count as "new," it must have been launched within the last 12 months of being identified (see box "Datamonitor's Product Launch Analytics Data Collection Methodology").

Attributes of new products are generally only incrementally different from existing products. Product introductions that closely resemble successful products may be viewed by companies as less risky compared to major changes since consumers are averse to radically different products (Padberg and Westgren, 1979). Datamonitor identifies six types of innovative new products that are the first to offer breakthrough features and benefits:

1. **Innovative formulations** include a first-ever variety or products containing new ingredients that offer benefits not previously provided. Examples include a tortilla chip line made from blue corn that contains fruits such as blueberries, strawberries and cranberries; a gluten-free chocolate glazed doughnut; and popcorn that is high in omega-3, omega-6, and omega-9 fatty acids.
2. **Innovative positioning** targets new users or positioning for new uses compared to existing products, such as a raw pork product geared exclusively toward making fajitas and a sandwich spread designed specifically for panini sandwiches.
3. **Innovative packaging benefit** provides a new benefit through package design, for example, a compostable bag for chips that is made from wood pulp sourced from tree plantations that are certified by the Forest Stewardship Council, a rice pouch that converts to a bowl, and a plastic bottle with a built-in straw.
4. **New market** products create a new market that does not compete with any existing product categories, such as a sandwich packaged in a can that offers convenience and protection for people on the go.
5. **Innovative technology** includes new products that use a new manufacturing process to provide consumer benefits. For example, advanced freezing technology for fully cooked rice that prevents the rice from clumping to allow the consumer to control serving size, and an innovative process that allows plant-based material to be used in

plastic bottles that replaces nonrenewable resources typically used, such as petroleum.

Datamonitor's Product Launch Analytics Data Collection Methodology

New product information for Datamonitor's Product Launch Analytics (PLA) database is captured from a variety of primary and secondary sources. The major primary source of data is actual new product samples. These samples are obtained through regular shopping trips conducted by PLA shoppers and staff, trade show visits by PLA staff, and samples sent by manufacturers and retailers. Regular visits are made to local retail outlets to purchase new products, including grocery chains, drug stores and pharmacies, convenience stores, club stores, mass merchandisers, hypermarkets, health food stores, and gourmet and specialty stores. PLA shoppers are asked to target specific categories and brands. PLA editors attend trade shows on a regular basis to gain first-hand information on new product launches, in some cases before the products reach the shelves. Through partnerships with key marketers/manufacturers, new product samples are sometimes sent along with a press release. Secondary data sources include company and trade websites, manufacturer and PR firm press releases, trade and consumer magazines and newspapers, and news and broadcast advertisements.

Data quality control measures include:

- Processes and procedures for data collection, product classification, and listing of product details,
- An editorial board to ensure consistency and quality standards,
- Intensive training of editors to ensure consistency across editorial offices,
- Stringent checks of all new reports before publication, and
- Checks of all product reports against past entries to ensure that that only new products are reported.

---

6. **Innovative merchandising** includes products marketed through an outlet unique to the category, for example, a unique display or packaging option, or a pouch of soup with a unique tracking code that can be used to track the ingredients and allows the consumer to see where each ingredient is sourced.

Typically, fewer than 10 percent of new food and beverage product introductions are classified by Datamonitor as innovative. For example, in 2010, only 2.7 percent were classified as innovative, down from 7.4 percent in 2001 and 8.4 percent in 1995. Innovative formulations were by far the most common type of innovation. In 2010, they accounted for 80 percent of innovative products, followed by innovative packaging benefits (15 percent), innovative positioning (12 percent), and innovative merchandising (4 percent).[4]

THE USE OF HEALTH- AND NUTRITION-RELATED CLAIMS ON NEW PRODUCTS

We track trends in new U.S. food and beverage introductions with voluntary HNR claims over 1989 to 2010. We trace changes in food producers' use of claims after implementation of the NLEA in 1994, along with recent developments in claim usage. HNR claims include those from the list of most common claims/tags in the Product Launch Analytics (PLA) database. Because the number of new products introduced varies from year to year, the importance of HNR claims is measured by the percentage of new products with these claims.

In general, between 25 percent and 44 percent of new products carried at least one HNR claim on an annual basis from 1989 to 2010. Use of the claims displayed divergent trends over the period (fig. 1). From 1989 to 2001, the percentage of new products with at least one HNR claim trended downward, from 34.6 percent in 1989 to 25.2 percent in 2001. After 2001, this percentage showed a marked reversal from earlier years, increasing from 25.2 percent in 2001 to 43.1 percent in 2010.

In the following sections, we delineate HNR claims by food categories and type of nutrient claims to gain insight into the underlying factors associated with the general trends described earlier in this report. We trace changes in the use of HNR claims when use was declining (1989-2001) and when it was growing (2001-2010).

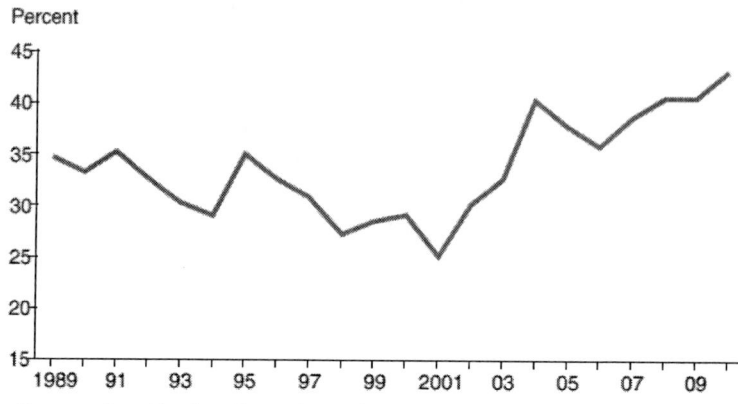

Source: Datamonitor, Product Launch Analytics database.

Figure 1. Percentage of new food and beverage products with health- and nutrition-related claims, 1989-2010.

NEW FOOD LABELING REGULATIONS AND USE OF HEALTH- AND NUTRITION-RELATED CLAIMS FROM 1989 AND 2001

The downward trend in new product introductions with HNR claims over 1989 to 2001 suggests that implementation of the NLEA in 1994 may have restricted use of the claims. This corroborates an earlier analysis of existing products at a representative superstore by Caswell et al. (2003). They found that the percentage of products with voluntary health and nutrient content claims fell by 5 percentage points from 1992 to 1999. As noted by Caswell et al. (2003), the impact of NLEA on voluntary nutrient content claims may be understated in their study if manufacturers began to adjust to the new regulations prior to their implementation.[5]

For those products with HNR claims, the number of claims per product increased from 2.0 claims in 1989 to 2.2 in 2001. This lends support for the "unfolding hypothesis," that competition between companies will lead to a more complete representation of the nutrition and health dimensions of their products than provided through a single claim (Ippolito and Mathios, 1994; Ippolito and Pappalardo, 2002). The NLEA did not appear to undermine the unfolding process, but may have contributed to its expansion by providing a credible means of promoting the health and nutritional characteristics of products.

Health and Nutrition-Related Claims by Food Category

Appendix 1 table 1 shows the percentage of new products with HNR claims in 16 product categories and several subcategories in select years from 1989 to 2010. Over 1989 to 2001, the percentage of products that carried HNR claims fell in 12 of the 16 categories. Oils and fats, such as cooking spray, shortening, and frying oil, had by far the largest reduction, falling from 65.8 percent to 19.6 percent. Ippolito and Pappalardo (2002) found that after publication of proposed NLEA regulations in 1991, which prohibit health claims for products that are not low fat, health and nutritional claims in the oils and fats category fell dramatically. This suggests that the NLEA rules may have shifted the focus of competition in the oils and fats category away from nutrition to other issues.[6] Reductions in the other 11 categories ranged from 0.6 percentage points for beverages to 15 percentage points, led by desserts and ice cream (-14.4 points); meat, fish, and poultry (-13.9 points); bakery items (-12.6 points); and snacks (-11.4 points) (fig. 2). Declines in the bakery, snack, and oils and fats categories occurred prior to 1994, perhaps in anticipation of the NLEA.

Four categories had relatively modest percentage point increases in HNR claims, including fruits and vegetables (4.7 points), soup (2.4 points), baby food (1.9 points), and meals and entrees (1.5 points).[7] Hence, following NLEA, there was some redistribution of HNR claims from products such as oils and fats, desserts and ice cream, bakery items, and snacks toward meals and entrees, soup, and fruits and vegetables. This suggests that the post-NLEA environment was successful in inducing greater health focus in advertising for the foods targeted for increased consumption, such as fruit and vegetables, compared to foods targeted for reduced consumption, such as fats and oils. Caswell et al. (2003) also found redistribution of nutrient content claims away from products such as oils and cookies and toward soups and vegetables, based on products sold at a superstore. Lohman and Kant (1998) surmised that after release of the Food Guide Pyramid in 1992, the frequency of advertisements bearing nutrition claims would be expected to decrease for beverages, fats and oils, and sweets, and increase for fruits and vegetables. The 1992 Food Guide Pyramid emphasized eating fewer foods that are high in sugar, including sweet desserts and soft drinks, eating more fruits and vegetables, and using fats and oils sparingly (U.S. Department of Agriculture, 1992).

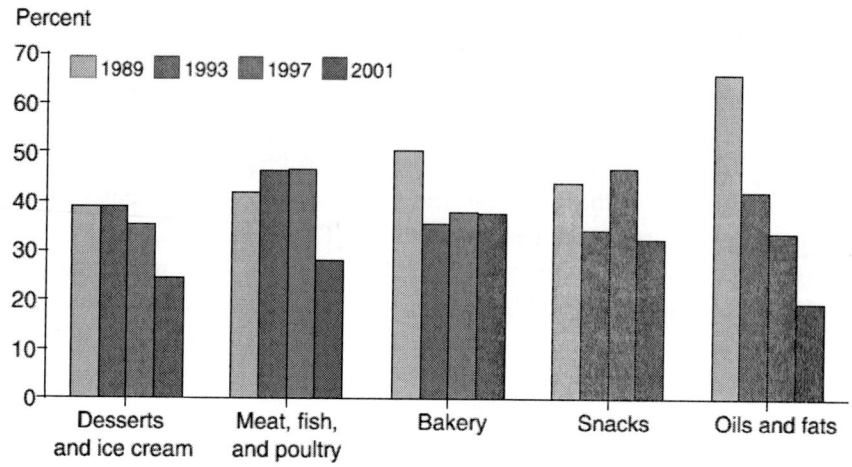

Source: Datamonitor, Product Launch Analytics database.

Figure 2. Percentage of new products with health- and nutrition-related claims, by product category, 1989, 1993, 1997, and 2001.

Types of Health- and Nutrition-Related Claims

For the 19 leading HNR claims used over 1989 to 2010, the percentage of new products bearing the claims are shown in appendix 1 table 2. Low/no fat accounted for the largest share of new products (13.6 percent), outpacing high vitamins/minerals by 5 percentage points. However, there was considerable variation in the importance of specific claims over time.

From 1989 to 2001, five claims had sizeable percentage point reductions in percent of new products carrying the claim, including cholesterol (-10.4 points), sodium (-9.0 points), calories (-7.4 points), fiber (-6.3 points), and sugar (-3.2 points) (fig. 3).[8] Each of the five nutrients is required to be listed on the Nutrition Facts label, and conditions under which products qualify for nutrient-content claims are specifically defined. In addition, except for calories, FDA has established specific requirements for claims made about the health benefits of the nutrients (U.S. Department of Health and Human Services, 2009). The Nutrition Facts label is a potentially important source of background information available to consumers to assess nutrient and health claims (Ippolito and Mathios, 1993). For each of the five claims, reductions in the percentage of new products with the claims appear more pronounced prior to 1994, as the deadline for complying with the NLEA approached (see fig. 3).

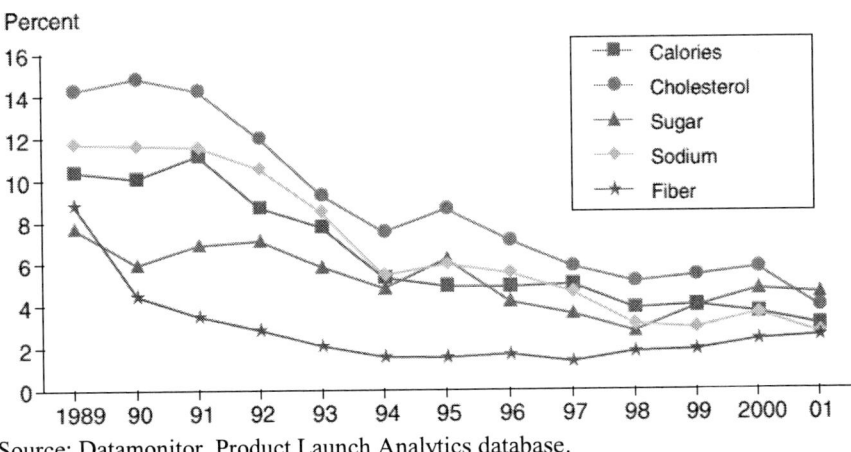

Source: Datamonitor, Product Launch Analytics database.

Figure 3. Percentage of products with health- and nutrition-related claims, 1989-2001.

These results are consistent with analysis of nutrient content claims in magazine ads by Ippolito and Pappalardo (2002). From 1991 to 1997, they found that the share of food ads with cholesterol content claims decreased from 24.7 percent to 5.8 percent. They also found systematic reductions in sodium, sugar, and calorie claims.

Food industry concerns that consumers associated poor taste with low- and reduced-sodium foods may also have contributed to the decrease in the percentage of new products carrying such claims (IOM, 2010). The industry has used two approaches to reduce sodium content through reformulation of existing products (IOM, 2010). The first is to change the sodium content of foods so that they qualify for sodium claims and market them to consumers interested in low-sodium foods. The second approach is to make gradual reductions in the sodium content of foods that go unadvertised, which is commonly referred to as "silent reductions." This is intended to allow consumers to slowly adjust their taste preferences for salt in the product. Neither approach appears to be widespread given the reduction in sodium-related claims and modest reductions in the sodium content across the food supply (IOM, 2010). Research to find replacements for sodium have not been as successful as some other nutrients, such as sugar.[9]

Eleven claims displayed percentage-point increases over 1989 to 2001, including vitamins and minerals (8.3 points), followed by protein (3.7 points) and calcium (3.2 points). Increases in the other 8 claims were each less than 2 percentage points.

Top Five Food Categories for Leading Health- and Nutrition-Related Claims

We evaluate the top five food categories for each of the top 10 HNR claims in 1989, 2001, and 2010. Appendix 2 table 1 shows the top five product categories contributing to each claim. Appendix 2 table 2 illustrates the top five product categories in terms of the share of new products carrying the claim to gauge their importance within a food category.

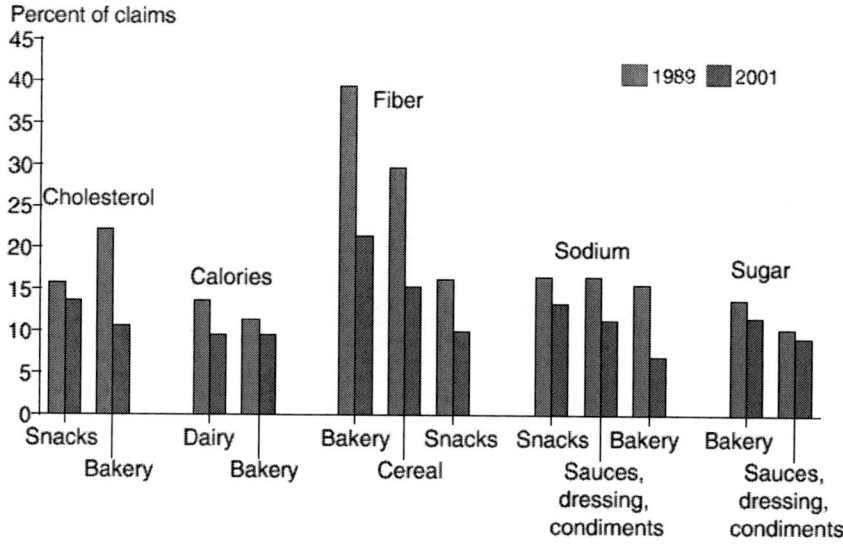

Source: Datamonitor, Product Launch Analytics database.

Figure 4. Product categories accounting for a smaller share of health- and nutrition-related claims from 1989 to 2001.

From 1989 to 2001, bakery products were important contributors to reductions found in the use of cholesterol-, sodium-, calorie-, fiber-, and sugar-related claims (fig. 4). Percentage point reductions were especially notable for fiber- (-17.9 points), cholesterol-(-11.5 points), and sodium-related claims (-8.7 points). The reduction in fiber claims carried by breakfast cereal (-14.2 points) was also prominent. In addition, cereal also dropped from the top five food categories making cholesterol-, sodium-, and sugar-related claims.

Snacks and sauces, dressings, and condiments accounted for a smaller percentage of three of the five HNR claims. For snacks, these nutrients included fiber (-6.2 points), sodium (-3.1 points), and cholesterol (-2.1 points).

Sauces, dressings, and condiments accounted for a smaller share of sodium- (-5.2 points) and sugar-related claims (-1.1 points) and also fell from the top five categories making calorie-related claims.

In 1989, bakery items, breakfast cereal, and snacks ranked among the leaders in the share of new products with cholesterol-, sodium-, fiber-, or sugar-related claims (appendix 2 table 2). Consistent with the findings above, these claims became a less important component of new products introduced in the categories from 1989 to 2001. Percentage-point reductions ranged from 3.2 points for sugar claims on bakery products to 47.3 points for fiber claims carried by cereal, which appeared on nearly 70 percent of all new cereal products in 1989.

GROWTH IN HEALTH- AND NUTRITION-RELATED CLAIMS FROM 2001 TO 2010

From 2001 to 2010, companies relied on HNR claims to a greater extent to market their new products in all product categories (appendix 1 table 1). Breakfast cereals had the largest percentage-point increase (30.1 points). Five categories had increases between 20 and 30 percentage points, including soups (27.5); snacks (26.5); sweet and savory spreads (22.7); meals and entrees (22.0); and pasta, pizza, noodles, and rice (20.6). The remaining 10 categories had increases ranging from 8 percentage points for dairy to 19.6 points for meat, fish, and poultry.

In 2010, breakfast cereal had by far the highest percentage of products with at least one HNR claim in 2010 (90.5 percent). Since cereals are usually sold in large boxes, cereal producers have a relatively low-cost means of highlighting the health and nutritional benefits on the package (Ippolito and Mathios, 1990). Many cereal marketers also have large budgets for advertising and product development. Other categories most likely to carry HNR claims in 2010 included snacks (59 percent), dairy (54.8 percent), soup (54.5 percent), and bakery items (50.9 percent). For subcategories, meat substitutes (93.8 percent), milk (92.2 percent), and yogurt (90.9 percent) ranked among the leaders in HNR claim usage in 2010.

From 2001 to 2010, use of HNR claims increased for all claims except low/ no fat, high calcium, and low/no carbohydrates, each of which fell by less than 1 percentage point (appendix 1 table 2). Many consumers found the taste of fat-free and low-fat foods introduced in the mid-1990s to be unacceptable

(Putnam et al., 2002), which may have led companies to limit use of low/no fat claims in later years (see box, "Low/No Fat Claims Peak in the 1990s").

The number of HNR claims per product also increased from 2.2 in 2001 to 2.6 in 2010 for those products making at least one claim. This provides further support for the unfolding hypothesis and competitive pressures based on nutritional issues that led companies to highlight more of the health and nutritional characteristics of their products.

New Diet and Nutrition Information and Claims Targeting Weight-Conscious Consumers

The overall growth in HNR claims from 2001 to 2010 reflects increases in claims related to calories, vitamins/minerals, whole grain, fiber, and sugar (fig. 5).[10] The increase in claims related to calories, fiber, and sugar was a marked reversal from previous trends (see fig. 3). The increase in low/ no calorie claims, compared to a slight reduction in the use of low/no fat claims, is consistent with findings by Kiesel and Villas-Boas (2010). In an experimental setting at a major supermarket chain in 2007, they found that low-fat labels on store shelves significantly reduced sales of microwave popcorn, while low-calorie labels significantly increased sales. This occurred despite the World Health Organization's endorsement of low-fat product promotions to reduce obesity rates. They attributed the results to consumers having less favorable taste perceptions of low-fat products compared to those that are low in calories.

Low/No Fat Claims Peaked in the 1990s

The percentage of new products with low/no fat claims displayed contrasting trends from 1989 to 2010. New products with low/no fat claims grew from 9.2 percent in 1989 to over 25 percent in 1995 and 1996. In 1997, they accounted for 21.7 percent of all new products, far exceeding all other health- and nutrition-related claims (see table 1). According to Putnam et al. (2002), mandatory nutrition labeling and consumer concerns about fat prompted food manufacturers to sell lower fat versions of high-fat foods. This led to a modest decline in added fat consumption from 1993 to 1997.

In contrast, from 1997 to 2001, new products with low/no fat claims fell by 11.8 percentage points to 9.9 percent.

Many companies reformulated their low/no fat products in the late 1990s by adding some fat to improve taste (Putnam et al., 2002). Between 1997 and 2000, per capita daily consumption of added fats increased by 16 percent. Since 2001, the percentage of products introduced with these claims has apparently reached an equilibrium between 8 to 13 percent.

The above findings are consistent with other studies of nutrient advertising claims. Ippolito and Pappalardo (2002) found that after NLEA enforcement, total fat claims in magazine food advertising became the primary nutritional focus up to 1997, away from other major nutrients. Analysis of supermarket sales data by LeGault et al. (2004) found that products sold with total fat claims had the largest percentage point *reduction* compared to other nutrient content claims from 1997 to 2000-2001.

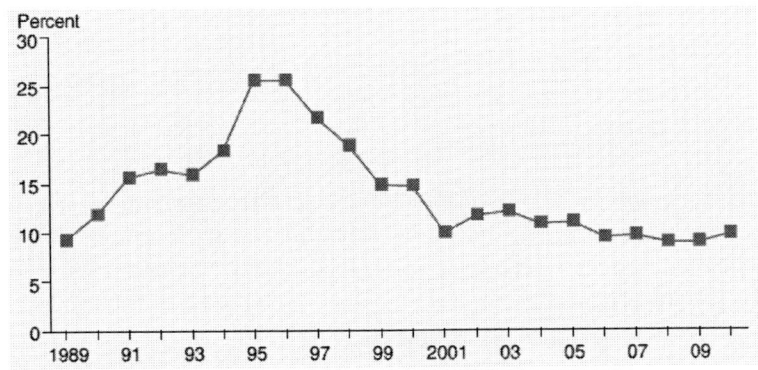

Source: Datamonitor, Product Launch Analytics database.

Percent of new products with low/no fat claims, 1989-2010 Percent.

The increasing emphasis on claims related to calories, fiber, sugar, and whole grain may reflect nutrition information from Government and nongovernment sources related to the obesity problem.[11] Statistics from the National Center for Health Statistics indicate that the percentage of obese U.S. adults and children increased from 1988-1994 to 2009-2010 (Ogden and Carroll, 2010a and 2010b) and Ogden et al. (2012). The prevalence of obesity among different age groups increased from:

- 22.9 percent to 35.7 percent for those 20 years and older,
- 10.5 percent to 18.4 percent for those 12 to 19 years of age,

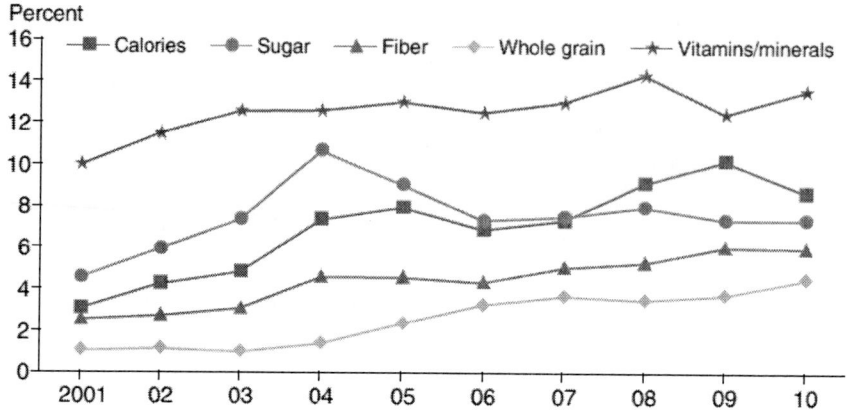

Source: Datamonitor, Product Launch Analytics database.

Figure 5. Percentage of new products with health- and nutrition-related claims, 2001-2010.

- 11.3 percent to 18 percent for those 6 to 11 years of age, and
- 7.2 percent to 12.1 percent for those 2 to 5 years of age.

In the nutrition area, information is usually disseminated through the release of Government studies or scientific panel recommendations and redistributed through the popular press (Ippolito and Mathios, 1990).[12] This, in turn, may affect consumer food preferences and/or product reformulations and voluntary labeling practices of producers (Chern et al., 1995; Golan and Unnevehr, 2008; Ippolito and Mathios, 1990).

We use U.S. national television network broadcasts related to obesity from 1989 to 2010 to gauge changes in obesity-related coverage. TV-News Search offers a searchable database of material in the collection of the Vanderbilt Television News Archive, which includes evening broadcasts and special news programs airing on CBS, ABC, NBC, CNN, and FOX News (added in 2004). Since the addition of FOX News in 2004 may have contributed to increases in obesity related coverage, rather than expanded coverage by existing networks, the network was excluded from our study.

The number of television news media reports from our search of headlines and abstracts using the keyword "obesity" increased after 2001 (fig. 6). In 2001, obesity was labeled as an epidemic by the World Health Organization (Gogoi, 2004), the Centers for Disease Control and Prevention (Seiders and Petty, 2004), and the U.S. Surgeon General (Gates, 2005). News coverage increased in the 3 succeeding years, with topics such as the National Health and Nutrition Examination Survey statistics on the cost of obesity-related health problems and how the food industry advertises sugary snacks to children. In 2010, news broadcasts rose to their highest level over 1989 to 2010. Thirty-six of the 58 news reports focused on childhood obesity (see fig. 6), including taxing soft drinks to prevent childhood obesity, the First Lady Michelle Obama's *Let's Move* campaign to fight childhood obesity, and the marketing of unhealthy "happy meals" to children.

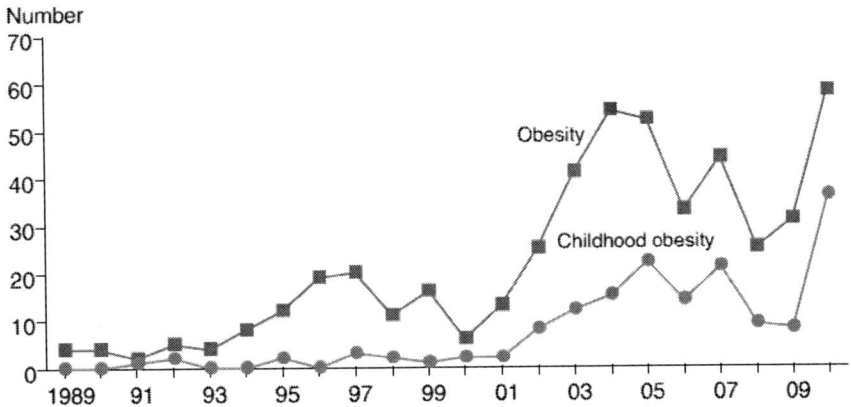

Source: Vanderbilt Television News Archive.

Figure 6. Television news reports related to obesity and childhood obesity, 1989-2010.

The Federal *Dietary Guidelines for Americans* may also affect the food industry's focus on new product development and marketing around specific nutrients related to weight control. The 2000 *Dietary Guidelines* recommended that consumers choose a diet to moderate consumption of foods containing sugars added during processing, which are often high in calories and low in vitamins and minerals.[13] Recommendations also included choosing a variety of grains, especially whole grains, to increase fiber, vitamins, and minerals. It was also the first edition of the guidelines to recognize the unique benefits of whole grains (*Dietary Guidelines for Americans*, 2000).

Key recommendations from the 2005 Dietary Guidelines included balancing calories consumed with calories expended, limiting calories by reducing consumption of added sugars, fats, and alcohol, and consuming a specific amount of fiber-rich whole-grain products (*Dietary Guidelines for Americans*, 2005).[14] New whole grain products as a percentage of all new products began to increase prior to 2005, most likely in anticipation of the release of the 2005 Dietary Guidelines and food pyramid emphasizing whole grains (see fig. 5). This occurred despite many consumers displaying no knowledge of the new guidelines or preferences for whole grain products (Golan and Unnevehr, 2008).

The whole-grain segment was expected to reenergize a stagnant cereal market, where sales were limited by the low-carb fad, growth in portable meals such as cereal bars, and lower cost private label versions (Lee, 2004). In 2004, General Mills, the Nation's second-leading breakfast cereal producer, announced that it would begin producing all cereals with whole grains (Horovitz, 2004). The move followed a Federal advisory panel recommendation that refined grains be replaced by whole-grain products to reduce risks of heart disease and other conditions. Following the General Mills announcement, Nestle announced a new Lean Cuisine line made with 100-percent whole-grain rice and pastas as sales of frozen meals were also limited by the "low-carb" craze (Thompson, 2004). Such product reformulations may also reflect efforts by manufacturers to improve their brand image (Golan and Unnevehr, 2008).

According to Mintel, a market research organization, the introduction of the Whole Grains Council stamp in 2005 was a driving force behind the rapid rise in whole-grain claims (Scott-Thomas, 2010). The Whole Grain Stamp program gave manufacturers the opportunity to signify the level of whole grain in their products as consumer recognition of the symbol increased. Companies must be members of the Whole Grains Council, file information about each qualifying product with the Council, and sign a legal agreement that they will abide by all requirements of the Stamp program. Such services strengthen the credibility of voluntary labeling (Golan et al., 2007).[15]

The growing popularity of low-carbohydrate diets also may have contributed to a surge in products with sugar-related claims, as consumption of processed sugars is discouraged in low-carb diets. The percentage of new products with low/no carb claims peaked in 2004, when it was the most popular HNR claim, accounting for 17 percent of all new product introductions (Datamonitor, Product Launch Analytics database). At the same time, the use of sugar-related claims also peaked, accounting for over 10 percent of new product launches. In 2004, 65.1 percent of products introduced with a no-sugar claim also had a low/no carb claim, compared to 5.7 percent in 2000.[16] By 2006, as the market for low-carb products had waned, the percentage of new products with sugar-related claims fell back to levels found in 2003.

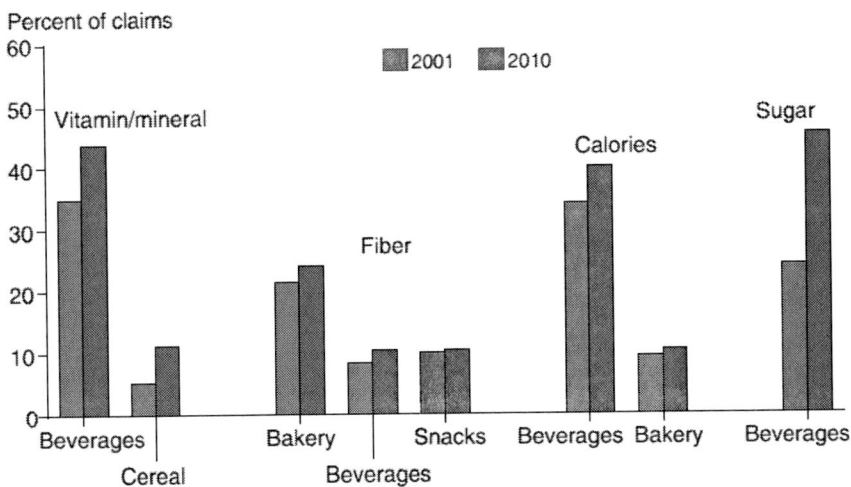

Source: Datamonitor, Product Launch Analytics database.

Figure 7. Product categories accounting for a larger share of calorie, vitamin/mineral, fiber, and sugar-related claims, 2001-10.

Sugar claims in the beverage category accounted for the biggest increase in the share of claims accounted for by a product category from 2001 to 2010, increasing by 21.3 percentage points (fig.7). In addition, there was a notable increase in the share of calorie claims accounted for by beverages. These developments followed the release of the 2000 *Dietary Guidelines* that emphasized the role of soft drinks and other sugar-sweetened beverages in the U.S. obesity problem. The 2005 *Dietary Guidelines* reiterated the need to limit calories from soft drinks and emphasized the importance of consuming nonfat and low-fat milk instead of carbonated soft drinks (*Dietary Guidelines for Americans*, 2005). Diet soda's share of the soda market grew steadily, as retailers gave low-calorie beverages more prominent shelf space to attract calorie-conscious consumers (Hirsch, 2004). Sales were also sparked by new flavors and sweeteners that provided similar taste compared to regular versions, but with fewer calories. While we cannot establish that growth in low/no calorie claims was due to the guidelines without industry corroboration, these results are consistent with those of Dharmasena et al. (2011). They found a statistically significant reduction in caloric intake from at-home consumption of nonalcoholic beverages following implementation of the 2000 *Dietary Guidelines*.

Snacks and desserts and ice cream moved into the top five categories with calorie-related claims in 2010 (see appendix 2 table 1). The growing importance of new beverage and snack products with calorie-related claims is especially relevant given that snacks and beverages between meals account for a quarter of Americans' daily calories (Scott-Thomas, 2011c).

Among calorie-, fiber-, and sugar-related claims, fiber claims in the cereal category accounted for the largest increase in the share of new products with a claim carried by a product category (see appendix 2 table 2). Thirty-eight percent of all new cereal products introduced in 2010 carried a fiber claim, up from 22 percent in 2001. This is a marked reversal from 1989 to 2001, when fiber claims carried by cereal products fell by 47.3 percentage points. Other notable increases included calorie claims carried by desserts and ice cream (11.6 points) and beverage products (9.8 points), and fiber claims in the bakery category (6.2 points). As expected, beverages moved into the top five categories with sugar-related claims, while snacks moved into the top five for low/no calorie claims.

Claims Target Evolving Consumer Needs and Preferences for a Healthy Lifestyle

While claims related to gluten, antioxidants, and omega-3 were used sparingly, if at all, prior to 2001, they ranked among the leading claims by 2010 (table 1). According to the Nielsen Company, products with "high omega-3," "high antioxidant," and "gluten-free" claims ranked among those HNR claims with the highest annual sales growth in 2009, increasing by 42, 29, and 16 percent, respectively (Pirovano, 2010).

Over 2001 to 2010, the percentage of new products with a "no gluten" claim showed the greatest percentage point increase among HNR claims, equaling 11.0 points (see appendix 1 table 2). By 2010, "no gluten" ranked second only to claims related to vitamins/minerals. The introduction of no-gluten products perpetuated sales growth in the category as companies responded to a growing number of consumers adopting a diet that is free from gluten— a protein found in wheat, barley, and rye. According to Packaged Facts (February 2011), a market research firm, sales of gluten-free products more than doubled from 2006 to 2010 and is expected to grow from $2.64 billion in 2010 to $5.5 billion by 2015.[17]

Some consumers purchase gluten-free products to control celiac disease, an inherited autoimmune condition that can lead to malnutrition, osteoporosis, and other potentially fatal health problems (Beck, 2011). Celiac disease has increased fourfold in the last 50 years and is estimated to afflict 1 in 133

Americans (Beck, 2011; Lapid, 2009; National Foundation for Celiac Awareness, 2011).[18] According to the University of Chicago Celiac Disease Center, 97 percent of those with celiac disease are undiagnosed. Gluten may also trigger an allergic reaction to wheat that results in hives, congestion, nausea, or anaphylaxis—an allergic reaction that may be fatal (Beck, 2011).

Table 1. Leading health- and nutrition-related claims for new food and beverage products in 1989, 2001, and 2010

1989		2001		2010	
Claim	Percent of claims[1]	Claim	Percent of claims[1]	Claim	Percent of claims[1]
Top 10 claims					
Low/no cholesterol	20.3	High vitamins/minerals	17.7	High vitamins/minerals	12.2
Low/no salt/low/no sodium	16.6	Low/no fat	17.5	No gluten	10.8
High fiber/high bran	12.5	High protein	9.2	Low/no fat	8.8
Low/no calories	14.8	No/low sugar/no sweeteners	8.1	Low/no calories	7.8
Low/no fat	13.1	No/low cholesterol	7.0	Low/no trans fats	7.7
Low/no sugar/no sweeteners	10.9	High calcium	6.8	Low/no sugar/no added sugar/no sweeteners	6.8
High vitamins	2.4	Low/no calories	5.4	High fiber	5.3
High protein	2.2	Low/no sodium/low/no salt	4.9	High protein	4.8
Whole grain	1.9	High fiber	4.5	Low/no cholesterol	4.3
High fruit	1.6	Low/no carbohydrates	3.4	Low/no salt/low/no sodium/ no added salt	4.2
Total	96.3	Total	84.5	Total	72.7
Other health- and nutrition-related claims[2]					
		No monosodium glutamate (MSG)	2.1	High antioxidants	4.1
				Whole grain	4.0
				High calcium	3.0
				High omega-3	2.2
				No MSG	2.0
Number of nutrient claim categories identified	17		28		36
Total number of health- and nutrition-related claims made	2,368		2,912		8,098

[1]Percent of all health- and nutrition-related claims.
[2]These claims accounted for 2 percent or more of all health- and nutrition-related claims. Source: Datamonitor, Product Launch Analytics database.

Surveys suggest that there are other health benefits that consumers attribute to a gluten-free diet. Based on a nationally representative online poll of 1,881 U.S. adults in the fall of 2010, Packaged Facts (February 2011) found that 15 percent reported buying or consuming products with gluten-free claims within the past 30 days.[19] Only about 10 percent of gluten-free consumers purchased the products because someone in their household had celiac disease or intolerance to gluten. The top reason given for purchasing gluten-free products is the perception that they are generally healthier (46 percent), followed by weight management (30 percent), and generally higher in quality (22 percent) (Scott-Thomas, 2011a). These findings corroborate an earlier nationally representative survey of 1,730 U.S. adults in July 2009 by The Hartman Group, a research consulting firm specializing in consumer purchase behavior (The Hartman Group, 2011).

Thirteen percent of respondents reported purchasing gluten-free products within the previous 3 months. Among these consumers, 5 percent reported purchasing gluten-free products to treat celiac disease. The top three reasons for purchasing gluten-free products were for digestive health (39 percent), nutritional value (33 percent), and weight loss (25 percent). Other health benefits ascribed to avoiding gluten found on the Internet and popular press include reducing the effects of rheumatoid arthritis, depression, autism, multiple sclerosis, osteoporosis, diabetes, attention-deficit hyperactivity disorder, and fatigue (Wilson, 2012; Scott-Thomas, 2011b; Solan, 2011; Gibeson, 2012; Gorton, 2010; Springen, 2008).[20]

In 2010, bakery items and snacks were the leading contributors to no-gluten claims (see appendix 2 table 1). Reformulation of products for the "no gluten" market presents challenges in some product categories. For example, removing gluten from cookies requires use of wheat-free flours, such as rice or tapioca flours, that may not provide the same texture and flavor (Wilson, 2012). In addition, alternatives to wheat flours may be deficient in protein, fiber, iron, calcium, and other vitamins and minerals (Gorton, 2011). Specialty ingredients are also more costly to source than wheat flour. As the demand for gluten-free food has expanded, companies have introduced new gluten-free products that overcome much of the sensory issues (Gibeson, 2012; Gorton, 2010).

The introduction and sales of products with antioxidant and omega-3 claims suggest that food companies were responding to consumer preferences for products that promote overall health beyond basic nutrition (Jones and Jew, 2007; Toops, 2008) (see box "Antioxidants and Omega-3 Fatty Acids: What Are They and What Do They Do?"). For example, an analysis based on

SymphonyIRI Group's (formerly Information Resources, Inc. or IRI) panel of over 55,000 households found that 60 percent are trying to eat snacks that prevent and/or manage health problems, while 24 percent seek benefits beyond basic nutrition (Wyatt, 2011).

A 2010 survey of a nationally representative sample of 1,579 U.S. primary grocery shoppers by the Food Marketing Institute and *Prevention* magazine found that omega-3 and antioxidants ranked among the top 5 ingredients sought by respondents (Scott-Thomas, 2011d). Factors driving demand for such "functional" foods include: scientific advances in understanding the relationship between diet and disease; increasing life expectancy and healthcare costs; and growing health awareness by aging baby boomers with monetary resources for slowing the aging process and managing chronic diseases, such as diabetes and cardiovascular disease (Archibald, 2007; Singletary and Morganosky, 2004; Roberfroid, 2000; Jones, 2010).

New Labeling Regulations for Trans Fats and Growth of "No Trans Fats" Claims

In 2003, FDA issued a mandatory disclosure regulation for trans fatty acids, or trans fats, on the nutrition label by 2006, which marked the first significant change to the Nutrition Facts label since the NLEA rules were finalized (Kozup et al., 2006).

Prior to the 1990s, there was little consensus from the scientific community on the harmful effects of trans fatty acid intake. In 2002, the Institute of Medicine recommended that trans fatty acids in the diet should be as low as possible and any intake was associated with increased health risk (Unnevehr and Jagmanaite, 2008). In 2005, the importance of limiting trans fats was further instilled by the *Dietary Guidelines* that recommended lowering trans fatty acid consumption to as low as possible.

Antioxidants and Omega-3 Fatty Acids: What Are They and What Do They Do?

When the body comes into contact with oxygen, a process called "oxidation" occurs, which can lead to permanent damage to cells and DNA. Oxidative stress may contribute to the development of numerous conditions, such as cancer, cataracts, arthritis, stroke, and heart disease.

Antioxidants are substances that absorb free oxygen molecules, which may prevent damage to the body that occurs naturally through aging (Gray, 2011; Archibald, 2007). Diets high in antioxidant-containing foods have the potential to improve overall health, delay of the onset of many age-related diseases, prevent eye disease, reduce the risk of some cancers, and improve cardiovascular function.[1] Some of the most common antioxidants include vitamin E, vitamin C, and beta carotene. In 1997, FDA amended regulations to define claims using the term "antioxidant" on labels, which became effective in 1999 (U.S. Department of Health and Human Services, 2008). The antioxidant nutrient must meet the general requirements for nutrient content claims related to "high," "good source," and "more." For example, for a "good source" claim, the food must contain between 10 to 19 percent of the daily value per reference amount customarily consumed per eating occasion (RACC). Omega-3 fatty acids are a particular type of essential unsaturated fatty acid. These fatty acids cannot be produced naturally in the human body, but are necessary for the body's metabolism. They can only be obtained by eating foods that contain them or by taking a supplement. Research has found that certain omega-3 fatty acids can aid cognitive function; prevent eye disease, depression, and muscle degeneration in the elderly; and prevent the incidence of cardiovascular disease (Packaged Facts, June 2011). A recent study of the mortality effects of 12 modifiable dietary risk factors in the United States found that having a low intake level of omega-3 fatty acids ranked among the top 3 dietary risks, behind intakes of high salt levels and ahead of high trans fatty acids levels (Danaei et al., 2009). Novel production technologies are now allowing omega-3 oils to be added to a greater number of food and beverage products (Packaged Facts, June 2011; Jones and Drew, 2007). In 2004, FDA approved a health claim for omega-3 fatty acids (U.S. Department of Health and Human Services, 2004b), which may have helped to legitimize and propel the market. According to Packaged Facts (August 2011), the number of consumers who are seeking high omega-3 products has increased dramatically over the past few years and will likely continue to grow rapidly over 2011 to 2015. Future growth is likely to depend on scientific data supporting its health benefits, new product introductions, and consumer awareness and demand.

---

[1] While the general benefits of antioxidants in the diet have been acknowledged, conclusive evidence does not exist for making recommendations concerning the consumption of certain amounts of antioxidants to combat specific diseases (Archibald, 2007).

As food companies revised labels to meet the impending 2006 deadline, some also reformulated their products with new trans fats-free oils and used claims to tout their lack of trans fats. Prior to 2001, Datamonitor identified no products with "low/no trans fats" claims. The percentage of new products with "no/low trans fats" claims increased from 0.1 percent in 2001 to 7.8 percent in 2005, which was the largest increase among leading HNR claims over the period (see appendix 1 table 2). From 2001 to 2010, the percentage of new products with "low/no trans fats" claims increased by 8.4 percentage points, which was the second largest increase among HNR claims, behind only "no gluten." In 2010, "low/no trans fats" ranked as the fifth most popular claim (see table 1). The increase in products with a "low/no trans fats" claim is testimony to competitive pressures in the food industry, as companies respond to new food labeling regulations and public communications that gave prominence to limiting trans fatty acids.[21]

In 2010, new bakery items and snacks were the leading contributors to "low/ no trans fats" claims (fig. 8). Growth in bakery and snack products with a "low/no trans fats" claim illustrates differences among product categories in the technical feasibility of reformulating products to contain healthier alternatives. Unnevehr and Jagmanaite (2008) compared oil ingredients used in new cookie and chip products with "no trans fats" claims to those introduced in earlier years. For new cookie products with "no trans fats" claims, partially hydrogenated oils—a source of trans fatty acids—were replaced primarily by palm oil or butter, which contain higher levels of unhealthy saturated fats. On the other hand, new chip products claiming "no trans fats" contained primarily sunflower, corn, or canola oil, which are healthier oil alternatives. While cake, doughnuts, and pastry were the biggest source of trans fats, few products were introduced with a "no trans fats" claim, which is also indicative of technical differences in the ability to find substitutes for partially hydrogenated oils (Unnevehr and Jagmanaite, 2008).

It is possible that companies who reformulated products to contain no trans fats following implementation of the new labeling regulations could compensate by adding unhealthy nutrients. Rahkovsky et al. (2012) found that among products introduced from 2006 to 2010, those that contained no trans fats did not have higher levels of saturated fats, sodium, or calories compared to new products with trans fats. In addition, among products containing no trans fats, generalizations could not be made about the healthfulness of products carrying a "no trans fats" claim versus those without the claim, since it depended on the nutrient.

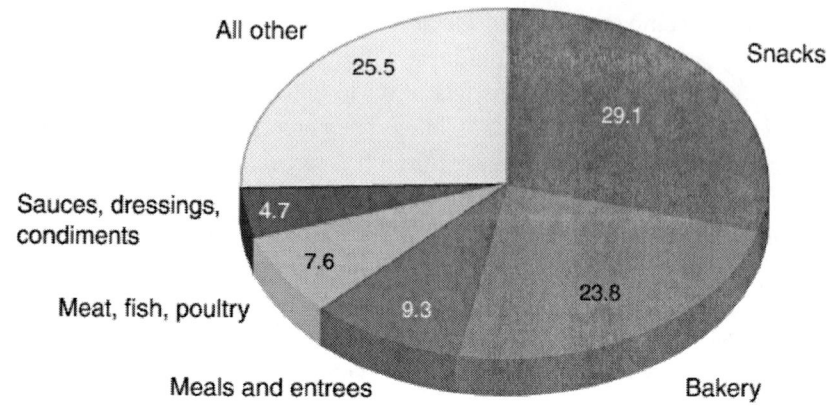

Source: Datamonitor, Product Launch Analytics database.

Figure 8. Percentage of "low/no trans fats" claims accounted for by the top 5 product categories in 2010.

SALES AND NUTRITIONAL CONTENT OF NEW PRODUCTS WITH HEALTH- AND NUTRITION- RELATED CLAIMS

The public health impact of new products will depend on whether HNR claims are effective in influencing consumer purchase behavior and the overall nutritional profile of products with such claims. Sales of new products with HNR claims provide some insight into whether these products are purchased and consumed. Because Datamonitor's Product Launch Analytics database does not contain sales data, this section compares sales and nutritional content of new products using market-research firm Mintel's Global New Product Database (Mintel GNPD).

New Product Sales

Mintel GNPD allows users to track new products carrying specific HNR product claims from June 1996 to present. Field associates shop for new products at supermarkets, mass merchants, drug stores, natural food stores, convenience stores, club stores, specialty stores, other independent outlets, mail order/Internet products, and some direct-to-consumer products. Mintel also monitors secondary sources for new product information, including trade publications, trade shows, company websites, press releases, and online newsletters.

The Mintel GNPD database includes information for five types of new products:

1. **New product.** New product is assigned when a new range, line, or family of products is encountered.
2. **New variety/range extension.** This launch type is used to document an extension to an existing range of products.
3. **New packaging.** This launch type is determined by visually inspecting the product for changes, and also when terms like "new look," "new packaging," or "new size" are written on the package.
4. **New formulation.** This launch type is assigned when terms such as "new formula," "even better," "tastier," "now lower in fat," "new and improved," or "great new taste" are indicated on the package. The ingredient list is not used to determine whether the product is a new formulation.
5. **Relaunch.** This launch type depends entirely on secondary sources of information.

Mintel partnered with SymphonyIRI Group to provide sales information for its new products. SymphonyIRI Group tracks sales of some products in Mintel GNPD at 34,000 grocery stores, drug stores, and supermarkets, with the important exception of Walmart stores, club stores, convenience stores, health food stores, dollar stores, and mail order/Internet products. The web-based tool for tracking sales is referred to as Mintel GNPD IRIS. Sales data are available beginning in January 2005. Tracking begins when a new product reaches 1-percent distribution (percent of stores selling). Each product record contains sales data for a maximum of 104 weeks. After this period, the products are no longer considered new, and sales are no longer tracked. The data offer only a limited view of new product sales because sales data are not available for new products that are:

- classified as new packaging, relaunch, or new formulation,
- private label (store brand),
- found outside of stores not covered by SymphonyIRI Group, as described previously,
- priced over $24.99, or
- not sold in at least 1 percent of stores.

We compare sales of new products with HNR claims to sales of all new products using Mintel GNPD IRIS.[22] Sales data are available for 27 percent of new products with the claims and 20 percent of all new products in Mintel GNPD because of the product exclusions cited previously. Average unit sales over 4-week blocks of time (i.e., quad weeks) are compared. Sales in week 1 (when the product reaches 1-percent distribution) are aligned for all products, and then tracked for up to 26 quad weeks (104 weeks).

We restrict our comparison to products that were introduced in 2009 and 2010 and that carry at least 1 of the top 10 HNR claims from 2010 (see table 1).[23] Sales of new products with nutrient content claims exceed that of all new food products, ranging from 8 percent higher in quad week 2 to 28 percent higher in quad weeks 18 through 20 (fig. 9). This suggests that products introduced with HNR claims were more successful compared to all new product introductions. However, because we do not control for other factors that could affect new product success, such as pricing strategies, packaging, advertising, and product positioning, our results only suggest that HNR product claims could be effective in generating sales.

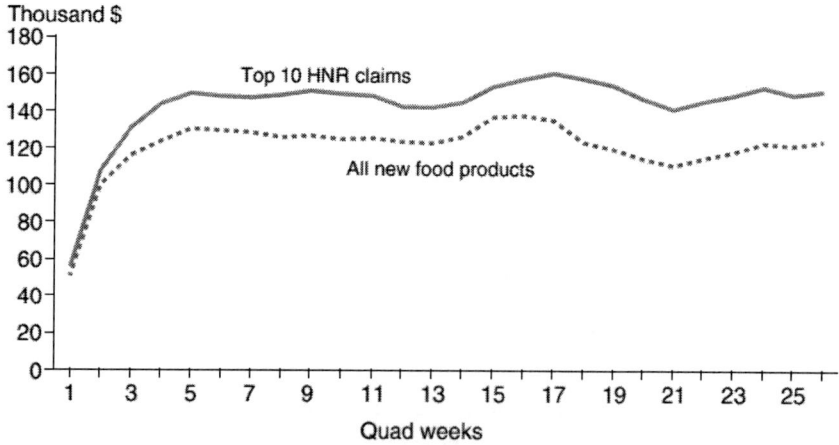

Source: Mintel, Global New Product Database IRIS (web-based sales-tracking tool).

Figure 9. Sales of new products introduced in 2009 and 2010 with health- and nutrition-related (HNR) claims versus all new food products.

These results corroborate findings from a recent study of Nielsen sales data from grocery stores, drug stores, and mass merchandisers by the Hudson Institute, a policy research organization (Hudson Institute, 2011). Nielsen data from 2007 to 2011 were first used to classify food products produced by 15 of the largest food and beverage manufacturers into traditional and "better-for-you" (BFY) product categories. BFY products are comprised of "lite" foods, or those designated as diet, lite, fewer, or zero calories (e.g., Lean Cuisine, Coca-Cola Zero, Tropicana 50), and "good" foods, including those generally considered as wholesome (e.g., whole-grain products) and healthier traditional product formulations that do not qualify as "lite" (e.g., Cheerios, Dannon Yogurt, Nabisco Wheat Thins). Traditional products, or those not considered to be a BFY item (e.g., Pepsi, Kellogg's Frosted Flakes, Hellmann's Mayonnaise), accounted for 61.4 percent of sales, while "lite" and "good" products each accounted for 19.3 percent of sales. While BFY products accounted for less than 40 percent of sales, they accounted for over 70 percent of sales growth between 2007 and 2011.

Nutritional Content of New Products

Producers have incentives to focus on the positive attributes of their products and downplay the negative. For example, Colby et al. (2010) found that nearly half of products with nutritional marketing claims (defined as any marketing, such as marketing on television, radio, or food labels, using health or nutrition information beyond minimum requirements) contained high levels of saturated fat, sodium, and/or sugar. This is of particular concern if consumers assume that products with HNR claims are healthier with respect to nutrients not mentioned in the claim ("halo" effect), or associate inappropriate health benefits to the product ("magic bullet" effect) (Roe et al., 1999). On the other hand, Ippolito and Mathios (1990 and 1991) found that competition among companies can lead them to improve multiple nutritional attributes of their products and market them by providing a more complete depiction of their healthfulness.

In addition to sales, we use data from Mintel GNPD to compare the average nutritional content of products with HNR claims versus all new food products.

However, nutrient content information is not available for some products when downloaded from the Mintel GNPD database. Not all products are required to carry a Nutrition Facts label. Exemptions include foods manufactured by small businesses and foods that provide no significant nutrition, such as instant coffee and most spices (U.S. Department of Health and Human Services, 2009).

Also, according to Mintel, nutritional information may not be available if the product is not acquired and secondary sources are relied on for new product information. In addition, if the product is a multi-pack item, nutrition information may not be available in separate fields for individual nutrients. Mintel cannot record nutrition information for multiple items on one product record since some products carry nutrition information for more than one component.

Over 2009 to 2010, we compare the nutritional content of new products with at least 1 of the top 10 HNR claims from 2010 to all new products. We focus only on products with no missing nutritional information. These products accounted for 64 percent of new products carrying a top 10 HNR claim and 56 percent of all new food products. Nutrient contents were standardized to a 48-gram serving to control for variations in serving size.

For each of the seven select nutrients that should be consumed in moderation, all new products had higher levels of the nutrients per serving, on average, compared to those with HNR claims (table 2). This suggests that companies did not use the claims to market products that are more unhealthy with respect to these nutrients. In addition, it suggests that if companies reformulated products to qualify for a HNR claim, they did not compensate by adding unhealthy nutrients.[24]

Table 2. Mean nutrient content of new products with a health- and nutrition-related claim versus all new products, 2009-10[1]

Nutrient	Unit	Top 10[2]	All new products
Calories from fat	Kilocalories	46.04	56.60
Saturated fat	Grams	1.54	2.34
Fat	Grams	5.16	6.34
Cholesterol	Milligrams	6.04	8.78
Sodium	Milligrams	205.84	253.42
Sugar	Grams	6.90	8.40
Trans fats	Grams	0.03	0.07

[1] Standardized 48 gram serving size. Differences in nutrient content are statistically significant at the 1-percent level of significance for each nutrient.

[2] Products carrying at least one of the top 10 health- and nutrition-related claims from 2010. Source: Mintel Global New Product Database.

CONCLUSION

The voluntary use of HNR claims on new food products is an important component of food companies' marketing strategy. In 2010, 43 percent of new food products carried at least one HNR claim. This compares to 25 percent of new products in 2001, which suggests that companies have increasingly chosen to compete by targeting health-conscious consumers. The extent of HNR claims on packaged food products introduced into the food supply highlights the importance of understanding how consumers use these claims, in conjunction with nutrition information, to form product evaluations.

Tracking of HNR claims beginning in 1989 reveals that the recent growth in HNR claims stands in marked contrast to reductions found in earlier years. From 1989 to 2001, the percentage of new products with HNR claims fell from 34.6 to 25.2 percent. This followed passage of the Nutrition Labeling and Education Act of 1990 that led to dramatic changes in food labeling by requiring most food products to carry a Nutrition Facts label and establishing rules for voluntary HNR claims. This suggests that the new food labeling regulations may have had an important impact on companies' use of voluntary claims and marketing messages conveyed to consumers.

The growth in "no trans fats" claims after 2001 lends further support to the importance of nutrient labeling regulations on the use of HNR claims. The biggest change to the Nutrition Facts label since NLEA (1990) was issued by FDA in 2003 and required food companies to include trans fatty acids in the Nutrition Facts label by 2006. The increase in new products with a "no trans fats" claim exceeded all other HNR claims from 2001 to 2005.

Claims related to calories, whole grain, fiber, sugar, and vitamins and minerals also were important contributors to the overall growth in HNR claims on new products after 2001. This followed communications regarding the obesity epidemic and educational campaigns by Government and other public information sources that highlighted the importance of calories, moderating sugar intake, and choosing foods high in fiber-rich whole grains. For example, the 2000 and 2005 *Dietary Guidelines for Americans* emphasized the role of sugar-sweetened beverages in the growing obesity problem and recommended limiting calories from consumption of such products. Sizeable increases subsequently occurred in the share of sugar and calorie claims accounted for by beverages over 2001 to 2010.

Other notable increases in HNR claims after 2001 included nontraditional claims related to gluten, antioxidants, and omega-3. For example, the biggest increase among HNR claims from 2001 to 2010 was for "no gluten," and it also ranked as the second most popular nutrient claim in 2010. The decision by food companies to feature these attributes reflects consumer needs and preferences for food products that provide health benefits beyond basic nutrition. Consumer demand for "functional" foods may be impacted by new scientific information linking diet and disease, an aging population, and growing health care costs.

Sales data for new products introduced in 2009 and 2010 suggest that HNR claims may have a positive impact on purchase behavior. This is consistent with the growing use of HNR claims by food companies and further highlights the need for understanding the implications of such claims for diet and health. In general, our study indicates that HNR claims not only highlight health and nutritional benefits for consumers targeting specific nutritional characteristics, but also that products with these claims may have a healthier nutritional profile. Competition among food companies, along with a credible means of highlighting nutrient and health impacts, may provide incentives to use HNR claims on products of higher nutritional quality.

REFERENCES

Allshouse, J., B. Frazao, and J. Turpening. 2002. "Are Americans Turning Away From Lower Fat Salty Snacks?" *Food Review*, Vol. 25, pp. 38-43.

Archibald, A. 2007. "Antioxidant Products: Nutritional Science and Marketplace Opportunities," *Prepared Foods Network*, June 11, 2007. Accessed May 5, 2011, at: http://www.preparedfoods.com/articles/print/105875/

Arsenault, J.E. 2010. "Can Nutrition Labeling Affect Obesity?" *Choices*, Third Quarter 2010.

Associated Press. 2005. "Gluten-Free Market Goes Mainstream," July 27, 2005.

Beck, M. 2011. "Clues to Gluten Sensitivity," *The Wall Street Journal*, March 15, 2011.

Brat, I., and P. Ziobro. 2010. "Campbell to Put New Focus on Taste," *The Wall Street Journal*, November 24, 2010.

Brecher, S.J., M.M. Bender, V.L. Wilkening, N.M. McCabe, and E.M. Anderson. 2000. "Status of Nutrition Labeling, Health Claims, and Nutrient Content Claims for Processed Foods: 1997 Food Label and Package Survey," *Journal of the American Dietetic Association*, Vol. 100: pp. 1057-1062.

Carlson, L. 2010. "Front-of-the-Pack and On-Shelf Labeling: Tools for Spotting Nutritious Choices at the Supermarket Shelf," *Nutrition Today*, Vol. 45: pp. 15-21.

Caswell, J.A., Y. Ning, F. Liu, and E.M. Mojduszka. 2003. "The Impact of New Labeling Regulations on the Use of Voluntary Nutrient-Content and Health Claims by Food Manufacturers," *Journal of Public Policy & Marketing*, Vol. 22: pp. 147-158.

Chandon, P., and B. Wansink. 2011. "Is Food Marketing Making us Fat? A Multi-disciplinary Review," *Foundations and Trends in Marketing*, Vol. 5: pp. 113-196.

Chern, W.S., E.T. Loehman, and S.T. Yen. 1995. "Information, Health Risk Beliefs, and the Demand for Fats and Oils," *The Review of Economics and Statistics*, Vol. 77: pp. 555-564.

Colby, S.E., L. Johnson, A. Scheett, and B. Hoverson. 2010. "Nutrition Marketing on Food Labels," *Journal of Nutrition Education and Behavior*, Vol. 42: pp. 92-98.

Connor, J. 1981. "Food Product Proliferation: A Market Structure Analysis," *American Journal of Agricultural Economics*, Vol. 63: pp. 607-617.

Danaei, G., E.L. Ding, D. Mozaffarian, B. Taylor, J. Rehm, C.J.L. Murray, and M. Ezzati. 2009. "The Preventable Causes of Death in the United States: Comparative Risk Assessment of Dietary, Lifestyle, and Metabolic Risk Factors," *PLoS Medicine*, Vol. 6.

Dharmasena, S., O. Capps Jr., and A. Clauson. 2011. "Ascertaining the Impact of the 2000 USDA *Dietary Guidelines for Americans* on the Intake of Calories, Caffeine, Calcium, and Vitamin C from At-Home Consumption of Nonalcoholic Beverages," *Journal of Agricultural and Applied Economics*, Vol. 43: pp. 13-27.

Drewnowski, A., H. Moskowitz, M. Reisner, and B. Krieger. 2010. "Testing Consumer Perception of Nutrient Content Claims Using Conjoint Analysis," *Public Health Nutrition*, Vol. 13: pp. 688–694.

Drichoutis, A.C., P. Lazaridis, and R.M. Nayga. 2006. "Consumers' Use of Nutritional Labels: A Review of Research Studies and Issues," *Academy of Marketing Science Review*, Vol. 2006. Accessed December 16 2011, at: http://www.amsreview.org/articles/drichoutis09-2006.pdf

Finkel, Y., E. Alonso, and P. Rosenthal. 2005. "Gluten-Free Food Labeling in the United States," *Journal of Pediatric Gastroenterology and Nutrition*, Vol. 41: pp. 567–568.

Ford, G.T., M. Hastak, A. Mitra, and D. Jones Ringold. 1996. "Can Consumers Interpret Nutrition Information in the Presence of a Health

Claim? A Laboratory Investigation," *Journal of Public Policy and Marketing*, Vol. 15: pp. 16-27.

French, S.A., M. Story, P. Hannan, K.K. Breitlow, R.W. Jeffery, J.S. Baxter, and M.P. Snyder. 1999. "Cognitive and Demographic Correlates of Low-Fat Vending Snack Choices Among Adolescents and Adults," *Journal of the American Dietetic Association*, Vol. 99: pp. 471-475.

Gallegher, J. 2011. "Survival of the Fittest," *Supermarket News*, October 24, 2011.

Garretson, J.A., and S. Burton. 2000. "Effects of Nutrition Facts Panel Values, Nutrition Claims, and Health Claims on Consumer Attitudes, Perceptions of Disease-Related Risks, and Trust," *Journal of Public Policy and Marketing*, Vol. 19: pp. 213-227.

Gates, K. 2005. "Stepping Up," *Supermarket News*, March 14, 2005.

Gelski, J. 2005. "Numbers Game Swings Low-Calorie Way," *Milling & Baking News*, July 5, 2005.

Ghani, W.I., and N.M. Childs. 1999. "Wealth Effects of the Passage of the Nutrition Labeling and Education Act of 1990 for Large U.S. Multinational Food Corporations," *Journal of Public Policy and Marketing*, Vol. 18: pp. 147-158.

Gibeson, A. 2012. "The Gluten-Free Quandary," *BakingBusiness.com*, January 17, 2012. Accessed February 1, 2012, at: http://www.bakingbusiness.com/News/News%20Home/Features/2012/1/The%20gluten%20free%20quandary.aspx

Glanz, K., M. Basil, E. Maibach, J. Goldberg, and D. Snyder. 1998. "Why Americans Eat What They Do: Taste, Nutrition, Convenience, and Weight Control Concerns as Influences on Food Consumption," *Journal of the American Dietetic Association*, Vol. 98: pp. 1118-1126.

Gogoi, P. 2004. "The Food Giants Go on a Diet: Rising Obesity Worries Force Big Changes," *Bloomberg Businessweek*, November 1, 2004. Accessed April 20 2011, at: http://www.msnbc.msn.com/id/6362472/print/1/displaymode/1098/

Golan, E., F. Kuchler, and B. Krissoff. 2007. "Do Food Labels Make a Difference?...Sometimes," *Amber Waves*, November, pp. 11-17.

Golan, E., and L. Unnevehr. 2008. "Food Product Composition, Consumer Health, and Public Policy: Introduction and Overview of Special Section," *Food Policy*, Vol. 33: pp. 465-469.

Gorton, L. 2011. "Niche Formulating: The Five Essentials," *BakingBusiness.com*, February 3, 2011. Accessed February 1, 2012, at: http://www.

bakingbusiness.com/Features/Formulating%20and%20R%20 and%20D/ 2011/2/ The%20Five%20Essentials.aspx

Gorton, L. 2012. "Ingredient Alternatives: Serious Concern," *BakingBusiness.com*, April 1, 2010. Accessed February 1, 2012, at: http://www.bakingbusiness.com/Features/Formulating%20and%20R%20and%20D/2010/4/Ingredient%20Alternatives%20Serious%20Concern.aspx

Gray, E. 2011 "What's a Calorie? (And More Nutrition Buzzwords Defined)," *The Huffington Post*, July 21, 2011. Accessed November 18 2011, at: http://www.huffingtonpost.com/2011/07/21/what-is-a-calorie. html#s 312674&title=Antioxidants

Harris, J.L., J.M. Thompson, M.B. Schwartz, and K.D. Brownell. 2011. "Nutrition-Related Claims on Children's Cereals: What Do They Mean to Parents and Do They Influence Willingness to Buy?" *Public Health Nutrition*, August 2, 2011.

Hirsch, J.M. 2004. "Calorie-Conscious Soda Drivers Drive Sales of Diet Products," *The Seattle Times*, December 22, 2004.

Horovitz, B. 2004. "General Mills Cereals Go Totally Whole Grain," *USA Today*, September 30, 2004.

Hudson Institute. 2011. *Better-For-You Foods: It's Just Good Business*, Obesity Solutions Initiative, October 2011.

Institute of Medicine, National Academies. 2010. *Strategies to Reduce Sodium Intake in the United States*. Washington, DC: The National Academies Press.

Ippolito, P.M., and A.D. Mathios. 1990. "Information, Advertising and Health Choices: A Study of the Cereal Market," *The RAND Journal of Economics*, Vol. 21: pp. 459-480.

Ippolito, P.M., and A.D. Mathios. 1991. "Health Claims in Food Marketing: Evidence on Knowledge and Behavior in the Cereal Market," *Journal of Public Policy & Marketing*, Vol. 10: pp. 15-32.

Ippolito, P.M., and A.D. Mathios. 1993. "New Food Labeling Regulations and the Flow of Nutrition Information to Consumers," *Journal of Public Policy and Marketing*, Vol. 12: pp. 188-205.

Ippolito, P.M., and A.D. Mathios. 1994. "Information, Policy, and the Sources of Fat and Cholesterol in the U.S. Diet," *Journal of Public Policy and Marketing*, Vol. 13: pp. 200-217.

Ippolito, P.M., and J.K. Pappalardo. 2002. *Advertising Nutrition & Health, Evidence from Food Advertising 1977-1997*, Staff Report, Federal Trade Commission, Bureau of Economics

Jones, B. 2010. "Prepared Foods Exclusive: No Functional Fad," *Prepared Foods Network*, February 2, 2010. Accessed May 26 2011, at: http://www.preparedfoods.com/articles/prepared-foods-exclusive-no-functional-fad

Jones, P.J., and S. Jew. 2007. "Functional Food Development: Concept to Reality," *Trends in Food Science and Technology*, Vol. 18(7): pp. 387-390, July.

Kaiser Family Foundation. 2007a. *Children's Exposure to Food Advertising on Television: A Side-by-Side Comparison of Results from Recent Studies by the Federal Trade Commission and the Kaiser Family Foundation.* Kaiser Family Foundation, Menlo Park, CA. June 5, 2007.

Kaiser Family Foundation. 2007b. *Food For Thought: Television Food Advertising to Children in the United States.* Kaiser Family Foundation, Menlo Park, CA. March 28, 2007.

Keller, S.B., M. Landry, J. Olson, A.M. Velliquette, S. Burton, and J.C. Andrews. 1997. "The Effects of Nutrition Package Claims, Nutrition Facts Panels, and Motivation to Process Nutrition Information on Consumer Product Evaluations," *Journal of Public Policy and Marketing*, Vol. 16: pp. 256-269.

Kemp, E., S. Burton, E.H. Creyer, and T.A. Suter. 2007. "When Do Nutrient Content and Nutrient Content Claims Matter? Assessing Consumer Tradeoffs Between Carbohydrates and Fat," *The Journal of Consumer Affairs*, Vol. 41: pp. 47-73.

Kiesel, K., S.B. Villas-Boas. 2010. "Can Information Costs Affect Consumer Choice? Nutritional Labels in a Supermarket Experiment," *International Journal of Industrial Organization*, In Press, Corrected Proof. November 26, 2010.

Kim, S.Y., R.M. Nayga, and O. Capps. 2001. "Food Label Use, Self-Selectivity, and Diet Quality," *The Journal of Consumer Affairs*, Vol. 35: pp. 346-363.

KPMG International Cooperative. 2011. *KPMG International Survey of Corporate Responsibility Reporting 2011*, Publication No. 110973, November 2011.

Koplan, J.P., C.T. Liverman, and V.A. Kraak, editors. 2005. *Preventing Childhood Obesity: Health in the Balance.* Washington, DC: The National Academies Press, 2005.

Koplan, J.P., C.T. Liverman, V.A. Kraak, and S.L. Wisham, editors. 2006. *Progress in Preventing Childhood Obesity: How Do We Measure Up?* Washington, DC: The National Academies Press, 2006.

Kozup, J., S. Burton, and E.H. Creyer. 2006. "The Provision of Trans Fat Information and Its Interaction with Consumer Knowledge," *The Journal of Consumer Affairs*, Vol. 40: pp. 163-176.

Kozup, J.C., E.H. Creyer, and S. Burton. 2003. "Making Healthful Food Choices: The Influence of Health Claims and Nutrition Information on Consumers' Evaluations of Packaged Food Products and Restaurant Menu Items," *Journal of Marketing*, Vol. 67: pp. 19-34.

Lapid, N. 2009. "The Celiac Disease Diagnosis Rate," *About.com*, April 1, 2009. Accessed April 13 2012, at: http://celiacdisease.about.com/od/diagnosingceliacdisease/a/DiagnosisRate.htm.

Lee, T. "Big G Takes High Road With Whole Grains," *Star Tribune*, October 10, 2004.

LeGault, L., M.B. Brandt, N. McCabe, C. Adler, A.M. Brown, and S. Brecher. 2004. "2000-2001 Food Label and Package Survey: An Update on Prevalence of Nutrition Labeling and Claims on Processed, Packaged Foods," *Journal of the American Dietary Association*, Vol. 104: pp. 952-958.

Levi, J., S. Vinter, L. Richardson, R. St. Laurent, and L.M. Segal. 2009. *F as in Fat: How Obesity Policies are Failing in America*. Washington, DC: Trust for America's Health, July 2009.

Lohmann, J. and A.K. Kant. 1998. "Effect of the Food Guide Pyramid on Food Advertising," *Journal of Nutrition Education*, Vol. 30: pp. 23-28.

Mancino, L., F. Kuchler, and E. Leibtag. 2008. "Getting Consumers to Eat More Whole Grains: The Role of Policy, Information, and Food Manufacturers," *Food Policy*, Vol. 33: pp. 489-496.

McLaughlin, E.W., and V.R. Rao. 1990. "The Strategic Role of Supermarket Buyer Intermediaries in New Product Selection: Implications for Systemwide Efficiency," *American Journal of Agricultural Economics*, Vol. 72: pp. 358-370.

Mitra, A., M. Hastak, G.T. Ford, and D. Jones Ringold. 1999. "Can the Educationally Disadvantaged Interpret the FDA-Mandated Nutrition Facts Panel in the Presence of an Implied Health Claim?" *Journal of Public Policy and Marketing*, Vol. 18: pp. 106-117.

Moorman, C. 1998. "Market-Level Effects of Information: Competitive Responses and Consumer Dynamics," *Journal of Marketing Research*, Vol. 35: pp. 82-98.

Moorman, C., R. Ferraro, and J. Huber. September/October 2012. "Unintended Nutrition Consequences: Firm Responses to the Nutrition and Education Act," *Marketing Science*, Vol. 31:738-755.

National Foundation for Celiac Awareness. 2011. *Celiac Disease Facts and Figures*. Accessed April 13, 2012, at: http://www.celiaccentral.org/celiac-disease/facts-and-figures/

Nielsenwire. 2010. "U.S. Healthy Eating Trends Part 1: Commitment Trumps the Economic Pinch," January 26, 2010. Accessed August 31 2011, at: http://blog.nielsen.com/nielsenwire/consumer/healthy-eating-trends-pt-1-commitment-trumps-the-economic-pinch/

O'Donnell, C. 2008. "Choices for Weight Management Products," *Prepared Foods Network*, May 2008. Accessed May 5 2011, at: http://www.preparedfoods.com/articles/article-choices-for-weight-management-products-may-2008

Ogden, C.L., and M.D. Carroll. 2010a. "Prevalence of Overweight, Obesity, and Extreme Obesity Among Adults: United States, Trends 1960-1962 Through 2007-2008," *Health E-Stats*, National Center for Health Statistics, January 2010.

Ogden, C.L., and M.D. Carroll. 2010b. "Prevalence of Obesity Among Children and Adolescents: United States, Trends 1963-1965 Through 2007-2008," *Health E-Stats*, National Center for Health Statistics, June 2010.

Ogden, C.L., M.D. Carroll, B.K. Kit, K.M. Flegal. 2012. *Prevalence of Obesity in the United States, 2009-2010*, Data Brief No. 82, National Center for Health Statistics, January.

Packaged Facts. 2011. *Gluten-Free Foods and Beverages in the U.S.*, 3rd Edition, February.

Packaged Facts. 2011. *Omega-3 Foods and Beverages in the U.S.*, 3rd Edition, June.

Packaged Facts. 2011. *Omega-3: Global Product Trends and Opportunities*, August.

Padberg, D.I. 1992. "Nutritional Labeling as a Policy Instrument," *American Journal of Agricultural Economics*, Vol. 74: pp. 1208-1212.

Padberg, D.I., and R.E. Westgren. 1979. "Product Competition and Consumer Behavior in the Food Industries," *American Journal of Agricultural Economics*, Vol. 61: pp. 620-625.

Parker, B.J. 2003. "Food for Health: The Use of Nutrient Content, Health, and Structure/Function Claims in Food Advertisements," *Journal of Advertising*, Vol. 32: pp. 47-55.

Petruccelli, P.J. 1996. "Consumer and Marketing Implications of Information Provision: The Case of the Nutrition Labeling and Education Act of 1990," *Journal of Public Policy & Marketing*, Vol. 15: pp. 150-153.

Pietzak, M. 2005. "Gluten-Free Food Labeling in the United States," *Journal of Pediatric Gastroenterology and Nutrition*, Vol. 41: pp. 567–568.

Pirovano, T. 2010. "U.S. Healthy Eating Trends Part 1: Commitment Trumps the Economic Pinch," *Nielsenwire*, January 26, 2010.

Progressive Grocer. 1997. "Special Report: Efficient New Product Introduction," July.

Putnam, J., J. Allshouse, and L.S. Kantor. 2002. "U.S. Per Capita Food Supply Trends: More Calories, Refined Carbohydrates, and Fats," *Food Review*, Vol. 25, pp. 2-15.

Rahkovsky, I., S. Martinez, and F. Kuchler. 2012. *New Food Choices Free of Trans Fats Better Align U.S. Diets With Health Recommendations*, EIB-95, U.S. Department of Agriculture, Economic Research Service, April 2012.

Roberfroid, M.B. 2000. "Concepts and Strategy of Functional Food Science: the European Perspective," *The American Journal of Clinical Nutrition*, Vol. 71, pp. 1660S-1664S.

Roe, B., A.S. Levy, and B.M. Derby. 1999. "The Impact of Health Claims on Consumer Search and Product Evaluation Outcomes: Results from FDA Experimental Data," *Journal of Public Policy & Marketing*, Vol. 18: pp. 89-105.

Röger, C., R. Herrmann, and J. Connor. 2000. "Determinants of New Product Introductions in the US Food Industry: A Panel-Model Approach," *Applied Economics Letters*, Vol. 7: pp. 743-748.

Sachdev, A. 2001. "New Food Products Battle for Survival," *Chicago Tribune*, May 8, 2001.

Scott-Thomas, C. 2010. *Whole Grains Claims Soar in 2010*, Food Navigator-USA, September 20, 2010.

Scott-Thomas, C. 2011a. *Celiac Disease May Have Little Influence on Soaring Gluten-Free Market*, Food Navigator-USA, February 4, 2011.

Scott-Thomas, C. 2011b. *Gaining Loyalty in the Gluten-Free Market*, Food Navigator-USA, April 4, 2011.

Scott-Thomas, C. 2011c. *Snacks Deliver a Quarter of U.S. Calorie Intake*, Food Navigator-USA, June 24, 2011.

Scott-Thomas, C. 2011d. *Fortification Drives Consumer Definition of "Healthy,"* Food Navigator-USA, July 25, 2011.

Silverglade, B., and I.R. Heller. 2010. *Food Labeling Chaos: The Case for Reform*, Center for Science in the Public Interest, Washington, DC.

Singletary, K.W., and M.A. Morganosky. 2004. "Functional Foods: Consumer Issues and Future Challenges," *Journal of Food Distribution Research*, Vol. XXV: pp. 1-5.

Siro´, I., E. Ka´polna, B. Ka´polna, and A. Lugasi. 2008. "Functional Food. Product Development, Marketing and Consumer Acceptance—A Review," *Appetite*, Vol. 51: pp. 456-467.

Solan, M. 2011. "Is Gluten Making Us Fat?" *Men's Health*, January 31, 2011.

Springen, K. 2008. "A New Diet Villain—Are Gluten -Free Diets Healthier, or Is It Hype?" *Newsweek*, December 3, 2008.

Stewart, H., N. Blisard, and D. Jolliffe. 2006. *Let's Eat Out: Americans Weigh Taste, Convenience, and Nutrition*, EIB-19, U.S. Department of Agriculture, Economic Research Service, October 2006.

Szykman, L.R., P.N. Bloom, and A.S. Levy. 1997. "A Proposed Model of the Use of Package Claims and Nutrition Labels," *Journal of Public Policy & Marketing*, Vol. 16: pp. 228-241.

Tanner, J., and M.A. Raymond. 2010. *Principles of Marketing*. Irvington, NY: Flat World Knowledge.

Teratanavat, R.P., N.H. Hooker, C.P. Haugtvedt, and D.D. Rucker. 2004. *Consumer Understanding and Use of Health Information on Product Labels: Marketing Implications for Functional Food*, presentation at the 2004 American Agricultural Economics Association Annual Meeting. Denver, CO.

Thompson, S. 2004. "Nestle to Roll Out Whole-Grain Lean Cuisine Line," *AdAge.com*, October 21, 2004.

Thompson, S. 2003. "Wal-Mart Muscles Marketers Toward Low-Cal Foods," *AdAge.com*, June 30, 2003.

Toops, D. 2008. "The Year's Top-Selling Food Products," *FoodProcessing.com*, May 2, 2008. Accessed May 26 2011, at: http://www.foodprocessing.com/articles/2008/119.html

Unnevehr, L.J., and E. Jagmanaite. 2008. "Getting Rid of Trans Fats in the U.S. Diet: Policies, Incentives, and Progress," *Food Policy*, Vol. 33: pp. 497-503.

U.S. Department of Agriculture. Center for Nutrition Policy and Promotion. 1992. *The Food Guide Pyramid*, Home and Garden Bulletin Number 252.

U.S. Department of Agriculture and U.S. Department of Health and Human Services. 2000. *Dietary Guidelines for Americans, 2000*, U.S. Government Printing Office, Washington, DC.

U.S. Department of Agriculture and U.S. Department of Health and Human Services. 2005. *Dietary Guidelines for Americans, 2005*, U.S. Government Printing Office, Washington, DC.

U.S. Department of Health and Human Services, Food and Drug Administration. 2004a. *Calories Count: Report of the Working Group on Obesity*. 2004.

U.S. Department of Health and Human Services, Food and Drug Administration. 2004b. *FDA Announces Qualified Health Claims for Omega-3 Fatty Acids*, FDA News Release, September 8, 2004. Accessed February 9, 2012, at: http://www.fda.gov/NewsEvents/Newsroom/Press Announce ments/2004/ucm108351.htm

U.S. Department of Health and Human Services, Food and Drug Administration. 2006. *Draft Guidance: Whole Grain Label Statements*, February 17, 2006. Accessed January 19, 2011, at: http://www.fda.gov/Food/GuidanceComplianceRegulatoryInformation/GuidanceDocuments/FoodLabelingNutrition/ucm059088.htm

U.S. Department of Health and Human Services, Food and Drug Administration. 2011. *FDA Reopens Comment Period on Proposed "Gluten-free" Food Labeling Rule*, FDA News Release, August 2, 2011. Accessed December 8, 2011, at: http://www.fda.gov/NewsEvents/Newsroom/PressAnnouncements/ucm265838.htm

U.S. Department of Health and Human Services, Food and Drug Administration. 2008. *Guidance for Industry: Food Labeling; Nutrient Content Claims; Definition for "High Potency" and Definition for "Antioxidant" for Use in Nutrient Content Claims for Dietary Supplements and Conventional Foods; Small Entity Compliance Guide*. July 2008. Accessed December 28 2011, at: http://www.fda.gov/Food/GuidanceComplianceRegulatoryInformation/GuidanceDocuments/FoodLabelingNutrition/ucm063064.htm

U.S. Department of Health and Human Services, Food and Drug Administration. 2009. *Food Labeling Guide*. October 2009. Accessed November 17 2011, at: http://www.fda.gov/Food/ Guidance Compliance RegulatoryInformation/GuidanceDocuments/FoodLabelingNutrition/FoodLabelingGuide/default.htm

U.S. Department of Health and Human Services, Public Health Service, Office of the Surgeon General. 2001. *The Surgeon General's Call to Action to Prevent and Decrease Overweight and Obesity*. 2001.

U.S. General Accountability Office. 2011. *Food Labeling: FDA Needs to Reassess its Approach to Protecting Consumers From False or Misleading Claims.* January 2011.

Van Camp, D.J., N.H. Hooker, and D.M. Souza-Monteiro. 2010. "Adoption of Voluntary Front of Package Nutrition Schemes in UK Food Innovations," *British Food Journal*, Vol. 112: pp. 580-591.

Wansink, B., and P. Chandon. 2006. "Can Low-Fat Nutrition Labels Lead to Obesity?" *Journal of Marketing Research*, Vol. 43: 605-617.

White House Task Force on Childhood Obesity. 2010. *Report to the President: Solving the Problem of Childhood Obesity Within a Generation.* May 2010.

Wilson, N.L.W. 2012. "How the Cookie Crumbles: A Case Study of Gluten-Free Cookies and Random Utility," *American Journal of Agricultural Economics*, Vol. 94: pp. 576-582.

Wyatt, S.L. 2011. *State of the Snack Industry 2010.* SymphonyIRI Group, 2011.

Yach, D., M. Khan, D. Bradley, R. Hargrove, S. Kehoe, and G. Mensah. 2010. "The Role and Challenges of the Food Industry in Addressing Chronic Disease," *Globalization and Health*, Vol. 6: pp. 1-8.

APPENDIX 1 TABLES

Appendix 1 Table 1. New products with health- and nutrition-related claims by product category, select years, 1989-2010

Product category	Percent of new products with a health- and nutrition-related claim						
	1989	1993	1997	2001	2005	2009	2010
Snacks	**43.9**	**34.2**	**46.8**	**32.5**	**52.7**	**61.0**	**59.0**
Potato snacks	57.3	44.0	54.3	25.6	64.6	79.2	71.0
Other snacks	36.8	30.6	44.0	34.4	49.5	55.9	54.3
Bakery	**50.3**	**35.6**	**37.8**	**37.7**	**60.8**	**54.1**	**50.9**
Sweet biscuits/cookies	30.8	33.5	32.5	12.7	33.5	42.7	40.8
Bread and bread products	64.9	31.6	30.1	35.9	64.3	51.5	51.6
Savory Biscuits/Crackers	57.9	42.3	52.8	31.0	71.7	59.2	48.3
Other bakery	78.3	66.7	61.9	78.9	85.6	68.1	61.4
Processed fish, meat, and poultry products	**42.0**	**46.2**	**46.5**	**28.0**	**39.9**	**41.2**	**47.6**

Product category	Percent of new products with a health- and nutrition-related claim						
	1989	1993	1997	2001	2005	2009	2010
Meat and meat products	40.0	45.8	40.3	18.3	29.0	26.3	34.0
Poultry and poultry products	43.2	50.0	51.9	16.0	34.8	53.2	60.0
Meat substitutes	71.4	73.9	87.5	70.3	81.8	94.4	93.8
Fish and fish products	25.5	13.0	21.3	32.8	51.4	41.0	40.0
Meals and entrees	13.0	13.3	20.5	14.5	32.1	38.3	36.5
Pasta, pizza, noodles, and rice	28.0	31.5	24.5	18.5	36.3	46.4	39.1
Sauces, dressings, and condiments	26.0	29.2	28.9	16.2	25.3	28.2	30.7
Dressings	49.4	40.5	52.3	26.3	50.0	38.3	46.4
Seasonings	26.7	33.0	23.8	13.1	24.8	21.1	27.7
Other sauces and condiments	18.8	26.2	25.7	15.2	20.6	28.8	28.5
Dairy	56.0	53.7	53.9	46.8	52.9	45.9	54.8
Yogurt	84.6	67.4	90.9	73.6	84.1	87.5	90.9
Milk	61.1	76.2	71.4	72.5	82.6	77.3	92.2
Cheese	34.6	31.6	33.0	19.2	31.2	19.2	22.6
Other dairy	68.2	63.5	58.3	48.5	58.1	51.2	45.8
Breakfast cereal	63.8	57.3	52.9	60.4	86.4	61.5	90.5
Chocolate, sugar, and gum confectionery	12.4	9.9	19.5	11.5	20.8	19.7	23.0
Desserts and ice cream	38.9	39.1	35.5	24.5	46.7	49.5	43.3
Beverages	26.4	21.9	19.4	25.8	33.1	39.8	44.0
Bottled water	57.8	34.3	28.2	40.7	73.9	56.5	50.0
Other beverages	23.1	20.5	18.6	24.5	30.9	39.0	43.6
Soup	24.6	40.9	51.2	27.0	33.3	54.4	54.5
Sweet and savory spreads	24.4	23.5	28.0	15.6	26.8	35.8	38.3
Fruit and vegetables	18.1	22.6	25.5	22.8	34.4	34.0	39.1
Baby food	9.5	22.2	12.9	11.4	20.8	23.9	20.6
Oils and fats	65.8	42.1	33.9	19.6	28.3	26.5	28.6
All food and beverage	34.6	30.3	30.8	25.2	37.8	40.8	43.3

Source: Datamonitor, Product Launch Analytics database.

Appendix 1 Table 2. Leading health- and nutrition-related claims on new food and beverage products, select years, 1989 to 2010

Claim[1]	Percent of new products with claim[2]												1989 to 2010[3]
	1989	1991	1993	1995	1997	1999	2001	2003	2005	2007	2009	2010	
Low/no fat	9.2	15.6	15.9	25.5	21.7	14.8	9.9	12.1	11.0	9.6	8.9	9.7	13.6
High minerals/high vitamins	1.7	2.2	1.9	2.2	3.9	6.5	10.0	12.5	13.0	13.0	12.4	13.5	8.5
Low/no calories	10.4	11.1	7.7	4.9	5.0	4.0	3.0	4.8	7.9	7.3	10.2	8.6	6.7
Low/no cholesterol	14.3	14.2	9.3	8.6	5.8	5.4	3.9	5.3	4.6	5.3	3.6	4.8	6.5
Low/no sugar, no added sugar, no sweeteners	7.7	6.9	5.8	6.2	3.6	3.9	4.5	7.3	9.0	7.5	7.3	7.3	6.4
Low/no sodium, low/no salt, no added salt	11.7	11.5	8.4	5.9	4.6	2.9	2.7	3.2	3.6	3.9	3.6	4.7	5.0
High protein	1.5	2.2	1.3	1.2	1.5	3.7	5.2	6.3	5.7	4.7	5.8	5.3	4.0
High fiber/high bran	8.8	3.5	2.1	1.5	1.3	1.9	2.5	3.0	4.5	5.0	6.0	6.0	3.7
Low/no trans fats	0.0	0.0	0.0	0.0	0.0	0.0	0.1	1.2	7.8	10.6	9.3	8.5	3.5
No gluten	0.0	0.0	0.0	0.0	0.0	0.0	1.0	3.0	4.1	5.6	9.0	12.0	2.9
High calcium	0.6	0.5	0.6	0.8	1.1	3.6	3.8	4.2	3.9	3.4	3.6	3.3	2.6
Low/no carbohydrates	0.0	0.0	0.0	0.0	0.1	0.4	1.9	3.9	6.5	1.5	1.7	1.2	2.2
Contains whole grains	1.3	1.0	1.0	0.9	0.5	0.7	1.0	1.0	2.3	3.7	3.7	4.5	1.9
No monosodium glutamate (MSG)	1.0	2.1	2.2	2.0	1.9	2.1	1.2	1.8	1.8	1.7	1.6	2.2	1.7
High antioxidants	0.0	0.0	0.0	0.0	0.0	0.0	0.0	0.1	2.9	4.8	5.6	4.5	1.7
Low/no saturated fat	0.2	2.0	1.2	1.1	0.8	1.3	1.1	1.0	1.3	1.7	1.3	1.2	1.2
High fruit	1.1	0.7	0.4	0.7	1.6	1.2	1.0	1.4	0.8	1.6	1.5	1.4	1.1
No/low lactose	0.4	0.5	0.7	0.6	1.0	0.9	0.9	1.2	1.4	1.0	1.4	1.8	1.1
High omega-3	0.0	0.0	0.1	0.0	0.1	0.4	0.8	0.8	1.8	2.2	2.5	2.4	1.0

[1] Includes those claims that accounted for 1 percent or more of all new products introduced over 1989 to 2010.
[2] Darkened line between the years 1993 and 1995 denotes pre- and post-Nutrition Labeling Education Act (NLEA).
[3] Includes all years between 1989 and 2010.

Source: Datamonitor, Product Launch Analytics database.

APPENDIX 2 TABLES

Appendix 2 Table 1. Top 5 product categories for leading health- and nutrition-related claims, percent of claims, 1989, 2001, and 2010

Top 10 claims in 1989			Top 10 claims in 2001			Top 10 claims in 2010		
Type of claim	Top 5 product groups	Percent[1]	Type of claim	Top 5 product groups	Percent[1]	Type of claim	Top 5 product groups	Percent[1]
Cholesterol	Bakery	22.2	Vitamins/minerals	Beverages	34.9	Vitamins/minerals	Beverages	43.8
	Snacks	15.8		Bakery	19.2		Cereal	11.4
	Sauces, dressings, condiments	10.4		Dairy	13.2		Dairy	9.2
	Dairy	9.4		Snacks	5.6		Bakery	7.6
	Cereal	6.2		Cereal	5.4		Snacks	5.2
Sodium	Snacks	16.5	Total fat	Dairy	18.6	No gluten	Snacks	16.3
	Sauces, dressings, condiments	16.5		Snacks	15.5		Bakery	15.1
	Bakery	15.7		Bakery	10.8		Beverages	15.1
	Beverages	12.9		Meat, fish, poultry	10.0		Sauces, dressings, condiments	12.6
	Cereal	11.2		Sauces, dressings, condiments	7.8		Chocolate, sugar, and gum confectionery	6.4
Fiber/branrelated	Bakery	39.4	Protein	Bakery	25.7	Total fat	Dairy	18.6
	Cereal	29.6		Snacks	14.2		Snacks	13.1
	Snacks	16.2		Beverages	9.3		Meat, fish, poultry	9.9
	Pasta, pizza, noodles, rice	7.4		Meat, fish, poultry	8.6		Bakery	8.7

Appendix 2 Table 1. (Continued)

Top 10 claims in 1989			Top 10 claims in 2001			Top 10 claims in 2010		
Type of claim	Top 5 product groups	Percent[1]	Type of claim	Top 5 product groups	Percent[1]	Type of claim	Top 5 product groups	Percent[1]
Calorie-related	Fruits and vegetables; meat, fish, poultry	2.4	Sugar	Pasta, pizza, noodles, rice	6.0	Calorie-related	Beverages	8.0
	Dairy	13.7		Beverages	24.1		Beverages	40.2
	Beverages	12.3		Chocolate, sugar, and gum confectionery	21.5		Bakery	10.4
	Bakery	11.4		Bakery	11.8		Snacks	8.2
	Desserts and ice cream	10.6		Sauces, dressings, condiments	9.3		Dairy	5.7
	Sauces, dressings, condiments	9.4		Desserts and ice cream	6.8		Desserts and ice cream	5.5
Total fat	Dairy	25.7	Cholesterol	Dairy	21.0	Trans fats	Snacks	29.1
	Meat, fish, poultry	16.4		Snacks	13.7		Bakery	23.8
	Desserts and ice cream	15.1		Bakery	10.7		Meals and entrees	9.3
	Bakery	10.3		Meat, fish, poultry	10.7		Meat, fish, poultry	7.6
	Snacks	7.4		Sauces, dressings, condiments	10.7		Sauces, dressings, condiments	4.7
Sugar	Beverages	19.3	Calcium	Dairy	36.5	Sugar	Beverages	45.4
	Bakery	13.9		Beverages	24.4		Chocolate, sugar, and gum confectionery	11.7
	Cereal	12.4		Bakery	16.2		Bakery	10.4
	Sauces, dressings, condiments	10.4		Cereal	3.6		Sauces, dressings, condiments	6.6

Top 10 claims in 1989			Top 10 claims in 2001			Top 10 claims in 2010		
Type of claim	Top 5 product groups	Percent[1]	Type of claim	Top 5 product groups	Percent[1]	Type of claim	Top 5 product groups	Percent[1]
Vitamins	Chocolate, sugar, and gum confectionery	8.5	Calorie-related	Pasta, pizza, noodles, rice	3.6	Fiber-related	Fruits and vegetables	6.2
	Beverages	26.3		Beverages	34.2		Bakery	24.2
	Cereal	21.1		Dairy	9.5		Cereal	13.9
	Pasta, pizza, noodles, rice	7.0		Bakery	9.5		Snacks	10.4
	Fruits and vegetables	3.5		Meat, fish, poultry	6.3		Beverages	10.4
Protein	Dairy	3.5	Sodium	Chocolate, sugar, and gum confectionery	6.3	Protein	Fruits and vegetables	7.4
	Meat, fish, poultry	45.1		Beverages	23.9		Bakery	20.8
	Dairy	13.7		Snacks	13.4		Beverages	18.4
	Snacks	11.8		Sauces, dressings, condiments	11.3		Meals and entrees	11.2
	Bakery	7.8		Dairy	10.6		Snacks	10.1
Whole grain	Sauces, dressings, condiments, pasta, pizza, noodles, rice	5.9	Fiber-related	Bakery	7.0	Cholesterol	Dairy	9.9
	Bakery	31.1		Bakery	21.5		Snacks	21.9
	Cereal	22.2		Cereal	15.4		Bakery	15.9
	Snacks	13.3		Snacks	10.0		Cereal	8.5
	Beverages	4.4		Beverages	8.5		Sauces, dressings, condiments	7.4

Appendix 2 Table 1. (Continued)

Top 10 claims in 1989			Top 10 claims in 2001			Top 10 claims in 2010		
Type of claim	Top 5 product groups	Percent[1]	Type of claim	Top 5 product groups	Percent[1]	Type of claim	Top 5 product groups	Percent[1]
	Pasta, pizza, noodles, rice, sauces, dressings, condiments; chocolate, sugar, and gum confectionery	2.2		Pasta, pizza, noodles, rice	7.7		Dairy	6.5
High fruit	Beverages	36.8	Carbohydrates	Bakery	26.0	Sodium	Snacks	15.8
	Cereal	18.4		Beverages	21.0		Beverages	15.5
	Desserts and ice cream	13.2		Snacks	12.0		Sauces, dressings, condiments	15.2
	Sweet and savory spreads	10.5		Chocolate, sugar, and gum confectionery	6.0		Bakery	13.2
	Snacks	5.3		Sauces, dressings, condiments	5.0		Meat, fish, poultry	7.9

[1] Percent of claims accounted for by the product category.
Source: Datamonitor, Product Launch Analytics database.

Appendix 2 Table 2. Top 5 product categories for leading health- and nutrition-related claims, percent of new products introduced, 1989, 2001, and 2010

Top 10 claims in 1989			Top 10 claims in 2001			Top 10 claims in 2010		
Type of claim	Top 5 product groups	Percent[1]	Type of claim	Top 5 product groups	Percent[1]	Type of claim	Top 5 product groups	Percent[1]
Cholesterol	Oils and fats	55.3	Vitamins/ minerals	Cereal	30.8	Vitamins/ minerals	Cereal	70.9
	Bakery	28.9		Bakery	23.0		Beverages	25.8
	Snacks	27.3		Dairy	22.1		Dairy	24.5
	Dairy	24.7		Beverages	17.9		Fruits and vegetables	11.9
	Cereal	23.6		Fruits and vegetables	14.8		Desserts and ice cream	11.6
Sodium	Cereal	34.6	Total fat	Dairy	30.8	No gluten	Snacks	22.6
	Oils and fats	28.9		Cereal	22.0		Soup	17.0
	Snacks	23.4		Snacks	19.9		Desserts and ice cream	16.3
	Bakery	16.8		Meat, fish, poultry	18.8		Bakery	16.0
	Pasta, pizza, noodles, rice	16.5		Soup	15.7		Sauces, dressings, condiments	14.9
Fiber/branrelated	Cereal	69.3	Protein	Bakery	16.0	Total fat	Dairy	35.5
	Bakery	31.6		Cereal	12.1		Desserts and ice cream	26.0
	Snacks	17.3		Snacks	9.6		Cereal	22.2
	Pasta, pizza, noodles, rice	13.4		Meat, fish, poultry	8.5		Meat, fish, poultry	19.7
	Fruits and vegetables	6.0		Pasta, pizza, noodles, rice	7.6		Soup	17.0
Calorie-related	Dairy	26.4	Sugar	Sweet and savory spreads	9.5	Calorie related	Desserts and ice cream	16.3

Appendix 2 Table 2. (Continued)

Top 10 claims in 1989			Top 10 claims in 2001			Top 10 claims in 2010		
Type of claim	Top 5 product groups	Percent[1]	Type of claim	Top 5 product groups	Percent[1]	Type of claim	Top 5 product groups	Percent[1]
	Desserts and ice cream	22.8		Desserts and ice cream	8.3		Beverages	15.2
	Oils and fats	15.8		Cereal	7.7		Soup	12.5
	Soup	13.1		Bakery	6.5		Dairy	9.7
	Meals and entrees	11.1		Chocolate, sugar, and gum confectionery	6.4		Snacks	8.3
Total fat	Dairy	44.0	Cholesterol	Oils and fats	14.3	Trans fats	Snacks	28.9
	Meat, fish, poultry	29.3		Dairy	14.0		Bakery	17.9
	Desserts and ice cream	29.0		Cereal	8.8		Meals and entrees	13.3
	Oils and fats	23.7		Meat, fish, poultry	8.1		Cereal	13.3
	Bakery	8.6		Snacks	7.1		Meat, fish, poultry	13.2
Sugar	Cereal	25.2	Calcium	Dairy	23.4	Sugar	Beverages	14.9
	Sweet and savory spreads	13.4		Cereal	7.7		Sweet and savory spreads	14.4
	Beverages	10.7		Bakery	7.4		Cereal	12.0
	Chocolate, sugar, and gum confectionery	10.1		Beverages	4.8		Fruits and vegetables	9.9
	Bakery	9.7		Baby food	4.4		Chocolate, sugar, and gum confectionery	8.0
Vitamins	Cereal	9.4	Calorie-related	Beverages	5.4	Fiber-related	Cereal	38.0
	Beverages	3.2		Dairy	4.9		Bakery	12.7

Top 10 claims in 1989			Top 10 claims in 2001			Top 10 claims in 2010		
Type of claim	Top 5 product groups	Percent[1]	Type of claim	Top 5 product groups	Percent[1]	Type of claim	Top 5 product groups	Percent[1]
	Oils and fats	2.6		Desserts and ice cream	4.7		Soup	12.5
	Pasta, pizza, noodles, rice	2.4		Meat, fish, poultry	3.7		Pasta, pizza, noodles, rice	10.0
	Fruits and vegetables	1.7		Bakery	3.5		Fruits and vegetables	9.3
Protein	Meat, fish, poultry	13.2	Sodium	Soup	9.0	Protein	Cereal	11.4
	Dairy	3.8		Cereal	8.8		Meat, fish, poultry	10.4
	Snacks	2.2		Dairy	4.9		Dairy	10.2
	Pasta, pizza, noodles, rice	1.8		Snacks	4.8		Meals and entrees	9.9
	Soup	1.6		Beverages	3.4		Bakery	9.7
Whole grain	Cereal	7.9	Fiber related	Cereal	22.0	Cholesterol	Cereal	19.0
	Baby food	4.8		Soup	6.7		Oils and fats	12.9
	Bakery	3.8		Bakery	6.5		Soup	12.5
	Snacks	2.2		Fruits and vegetables	5.4		Snacks	12.3
	Pasta, pizza, noodles, rice	0.6		Pasta, pizza, noodles, rice	4.7		Bakery	6.8
High fruit	Cereal	5.5	Carbohydrates	Bakery	6.0	Sodium	Soup	20.5
	Sweet and savory spreads	3.4		Snacks	3.0		Cereal	8.9
	Desserts and ice cream	3.1		Sweet and savory spreads	2.7		Snacks	8.6
	Beverages	3.0		Beverages	2.1		Meat, fish, poultry	7.6
	Fruits and vegetables	0.9		Pasta, pizza, noodles, rice	1.9		Sauces, dressings, condiments	7.0

[1] Percent of new products carrying the claim within the product category.
Source: Datamonitor, Product Launch Analytics database.

End Notes

[1] These claims accounted for 15.8 percent of all HNR claims tracked by Datamonitor, a market research agency, in 2010.

[2] FDA does not pre-approve all claims and, therefore, claims may be used that are not sanctioned by the regulations until they are challenged by the agency.

[3] An earlier FLAPS survey found that 38.7 percent of all products sold carried a nutrient content claim in 1997, and 4.2 percent had a health claim (Brecher et al., 2000). Based on analysis of food ads from three popular consumer magazines between 1998 and 1999, 65.9 percent of HNR claims were nutrient content claims (Parker, 2003). Structure/function and health claims accounted for 13.1 percent and 4.5 percent of all HNR claims, respectively. Caswell et al. (2003) found that more than 40 percent of sampled products at a superstore from 1992 to 1999 carried nutrient content claims, but less than 7 percent had health-related claims.

[4] Percentages do not sum to 100 since a product may have more than one type of innovation.

[5] They also contend that while consumer demand for nutritional attributes may also affect claim usage, demand did not change quickly in the mid-1990s, which is consistent with the conjecture that the NLEA did have an impact.

[6] Over 1989 to 2001, Datamonitor did not list nutrient content information to compare the nutritional quality of new products with HNR claims versus those without these claims. The most common oil ingredient used over the period was olive oil, which was contained in 55 percent of new oil and fat products. We flagged only 10 oil and fat products that contained oils with relatively high saturated fats or trans fatty acids, including coconut oil, partially hydrogenated oils, lard, meat fats, and vegetable shortening. Four of these products had claims of "low calorie," "no cholesterol," "low fat," "no trans fat," and/or "low saturated fat." While HNR claims declined over the period, claims of "upscale," "gourmet," "pure," "natural," "organic," or "no chemicals/additives/preservatives" remained central to the marketing of these products, ranging from 48 percent of new oil and fat products in 1992 to 85 percent in 1998.

[7] Between 1989 and 2001, soup showed considerable variation in the use of HNR claims, increasing from 24.6 percent in 1989 to 51.2 percent in 1997, before falling to 27 percent in 2001.

[8] Reductions in whole grain and high fruit claims were less than 0.5 percentage points.

[9] Recent advances in food science may facilitate further reductions in sodium content. For example, food science innovations enabled Frito-Lay to reduce the sodium content of its seasoned chips by 25 percent without compromising taste by cutting topical salt and other ingredients (Gallagher, 2011). The company chose not to advertise the reduction on its packages.

[10] For each of these claims, the share of new products with the claim increased by over 2.5 percentage points from 2001 to 2010. Sodium claims increased by 2 percentage points, with most of the increase coming in 2010 when they were carried by 4.7 percent of new products, compared to 3.6 percent in 2009.

[11] Increased emphasis on the obesity problem is also reflected by the formation of the Healthy Weight Commitment Foundation, which is a coalition of retailers (e.g., United Supermarkets), manufacturers (e.g., Kellogg, PepsiCo), nonprofit organizations, and trade associations formed in 2009 with the stated purpose of reducing obesity.

[12] For example, in 2004, an FDA obesity working group released a report identifying calorie content as a key nutrient in determining weight gain, and recommended giving calories more prominence on the food label (U.S. Department of Health and Human Services,

2004a). In 2005, the Institute of Medicine issued a congressionally mandated study, *Preventing Childhood Obesity: Health in the Balance*, to guide development of a plan to combat the growing obesity epidemic in children (Koplan et al., 2005).

[13] Another contributing factor to the growth in sugar- and calorie-related claims by manufacturers was encouragement from Walmart to introduce low-calorie and low-sugar versions of their products to counter flat store sales by targeting their more health-conscious customers (Thompson, 2003).

[14] Dietary fiber was important in the formulation of some companies' products that were targeted to consumers concerned about weight (O'Donnell, 2008).

[15] In 2006, the FDA issued guidance to the food industry about what the agency considers "whole grain" to mean, and to assist manufacturers with food label statements related to "whole grain" content (U.S. Department of Health and Human Services, 2006). The guidance contains recommendations that are not legally enforceable.

[16] Splenda, a no-calorie sweetener approved for use in 1998, was well suited for the low-carbohydrate fad and increasing interest in lower calorie and lower sugar alternatives. Based on a keyword search for the term "Splenda" in Datamonitor's Product Launch Analytics database, use of the sweetener peaked in 2004, accounting for 14 percent of all new products with sugar-, carbohydrate-, or calorie-related claims.

[17] In 2005, Walmart, the Nation's leading food retailer, introduced gluten-free products and required suppliers to identify whether gluten is used in its store brand products (Associated Press, 2005).

[18] In 2007, the FDA issued a proposed rule on gluten-free food labeling that foods bearing the claim cannot contain 20 parts per million or more of gluten, but a final rule has yet to be released (U.S. Department of Health and Human Services, 2011). In August 2011, FDA announced that it was reopening the public comment period on the 2007 gluten-free labeling proposal for 60 days.

[19] The sample was balanced to census data based on measures of age, gender, geographic region, ethnicity, and income.

[20] A strong body of scientific research that supports health benefits beyond that related to celiac disease and wheat allergy is lacking (Springen, 2008; Wilson, 2012; Solan, 2011; Gorton, 2010). However, a 2011 study provided scientific evidence of the existence of gluten sensitivity, or gluten intolerance (Beck, 2011). In this case, gluten can trigger a reaction in the intestines and immune system that is less severe than celiac disease. The most common symptoms include stomach problems, headaches, fatigue, and depression.

[21] According to FDA research, "no trans fats" claims by food companies increased despite consumers not knowing whether trans fats were good or bad in the period leading up to mandatory labeling (Golan et al., 2007).

[22] We were not able to compare sales of new products with HNR claims to sales of new products without the claims because of a glitch in the download feature of the web-based Mintel GNPD IRIS. Because users of the online database cannot access the disaggregated sales data, sales of products without the claims could not be derived by subtracting sales of products with claims from sales of all new products.

[23] Some aspects of relevancy are gone beyond a 2-year comparison, because new product sales data are no longer tracked after 2 years. We chose the most recent 2-year period and the top 10 claims in 2010.

[24] It is important to note that differences in the nutritional content of aggregate food groups will not necessarily equal nutritional differences in any particular food category. Results represent average nutritional content across all food categories.

In: Food Products Use ...
Editors: O. Chertok and M. Aberlieb

ISBN: 978-1-62808-440-5
© 2013 Nova Science Publishers, Inc.

Chapter 2

DO FOOD LABELS MAKE A DIFFERENCE? ... SOMETIMES[*]

Elise Golan, Fred Kuchler and Barry Krissoff

- Competition drives food manufacturers to voluntarily label their products' desirable attributes and to use third-party certifiers to bolster credibility.
- Mandatory food labeling is usually more successful at filling information gaps than at addressing externalities such as environmental or health spillovers associated with food production and consumption
- Mandatory labeling may initially have a larger impact on manufacturers' production decisions than on consumers' food choices.

There is a lot to know about the food we eat. The ingredients in a jar of spaghetti sauce, a box of cereal, or a cup of coffee could come from around the corner or around the world; they could be processed by children or by high-tech machines; they could be grown on huge corporate farms or on small family-run farms; or they could be mostly artificial or 100-percent natural.

While a description of a food product could include information on a multitude of attributes, not all of them are important to consumers or regulators. Information on some attributes could affect the health and welfare

---

[*] This article appeared in the November 2007 issue of Amber Waves, released by the U.S. Department of Agriculture, Economic Research Service.

of consumers by influencing their food choices. Information on other attributes might have no effect at all.

Consumers, food companies, third-party entities, and governments play a role in determining which attributes are described on the label. The interaction of these groups influences which information is labeled voluntarily, which is mandated, and which is not labeled at all. It shapes the way information is presented and the accuracy and credibility of that information. The economics behind food labeling provides insight into the dynamics of voluntary food labeling and the types of market failures best addressed through mandatory labeling requirements.

COMPANIES WILL VOLUNTARILY LABEL IF THEIR BENEFITS OUTWEIGH THEIR COSTS

Voluntary labeling is one of a food company's many advertising options. Assuming that companies attempt to maximize profits, they will add information about an attribute to the label as long as each additional message eventually generates more benefits than costs. The primary benefits of labeling for a company come from either increasing profits or maintaining profits in the face of new competition. Either outcome is more likely if consumers use the information to differentiate the labeled product from similar products and then buy it.

The probability that consumers will value and react to labeled information is improved if the label successfully persuades consumers that it conveys information about a meaningful distinction between labeled and unlabeled products.

If consumers decide that the information's significance or accuracy is questionable, they will not use it to modify their purchase decisions. Researchers from the University of California and ERS found, for example, that the geographic branding of Washington State apples is losing its impact because it does not convincingly differentiate the State's apples from those grown in other areas.

To bolster the meaningfulness of their message, firms often rely on advertising and other types of outreach. In 2005, the U.S. food industry spent $32 billion on advertising and $66.5 billion on packaging to differentiate their products from the competition (see "Food Product Introductions Continue To Set Records" on page 4 in this issue).

Firms may also try to convince consumers of the validity of their labeling claims by using third-party labeling services. By offering an "unbiased" assessment of a labeling claim, these services help strengthen the credibility of voluntary labeling (see box, "Third-Party Labeling Services Can Improve Market Efficiency"). A number of entities, including consumer groups, producer associations, private companies, national governments, and international organizations, provide third-party services. The Good Housekeeping Institute, for example, founded for the purpose of consumer education and product evaluation, sets product standards and provides consumer guarantees for a multitude of goods, including foods. Two private companies, Société Générale de Surveillance (SGS) and AIB International (originally the American Institute of Baking), verify and certify food safety for a wide range of food products. USDA's Agricultural Marketing Service (AMS) has developed official grade standards for meats, eggs, poultry, dairy products, fresh fruits, vegetables, tree nuts, peanuts, and other commodities. ISO, a worldwide federation of national standards institutes, promotes the development of international standards for a variety of products and production processes.

The value of the labeling service generally depends on the credibility and reputation of the providing entity. In some cases, national governments or associations of national governments may be the most widely recognized and reputable third-party providers of labeling services. But this is not always true. For example, although U.S. consumers tend to have confidence in USDA and the Food and Drug Administration (FDA) to regulate food safety, Europeans rank national bodies far below international, environmental, consumer, and farm organizations in terms of trustworthiness.

Private and government labeling services have helped support an explosion of voluntary food labeling. American grocery store shelves have become veritable encyclopedias of labeling claims. A single carton of eggs sold in a national grocery store chain, for instance, is labeled with a "cage free" claim, the grocery store "quality and satisfaction money-back guarantee" logo, the Orthodox Union symbol of kosher certification, and a long list of nutrient claims, including "25% of the daily value of vitamin E; 185 mcg of lutein per egg; and 100 mg of omega-3 polyunsaturated fatty acids per egg."

A byproduct of the explosion of labeled attributes is that consumers learn to "read between the labels" and make deductions about unlabeled products. For example, confronted with one can of tuna labeled "dolphin friendly" and one with no such claim, consumers would likely assume that the unlabeled tuna was caught with dolphin-endangering practices. In a competitive marketplace, the presence of a label is a signal of quality, and the lack of a label on competing brands implies the absence of the quality attribute.

VOLUNTARY LABELING MAY LEAVE INFORMATION GAPS

Economic theory predicts that voluntary labeling is not always sufficient for disclosing information on all attributes consumers value or for guaranteeing information accuracy.

One limitation to voluntary labeling may arise when an entire product category has an undesirable characteristic. In these cases, manufacturers do not compete on the attribute and therefore do not provide labeled or otherwise advertised information to consumers. For example, there was little information on the sodium content of processed foods before manufacturers were required to disclose it. The competitive process did not work well to reveal high-sodium products; few manufacturers competed to offer reduced-sodium products because less of this "health negative" attribute also tends to reduce taste.

Another limitation to voluntary labeling arises because manufacturers may provide only relative information. For example, a sausage label may boast "30 percent less fat than the leading brand" or a bacon label may brag "half the sodium." Although this type of information is valuable for deciding among competing brands of the same item, it is not complete. Lower fat sausage may still be a high-fat food. In many cases, consumers need information on absolute, not just relative, values to make fully informed consumption decisions.

Market forces may also be unable to eliminate partial disclosure and innuendo. For example, in early 2000, a manufacturer began marketing a wheat-flake cereal with a label proclaiming no "genetically engineered ingredients."

A consumer advocacy group asked the FDA to take enforcement action against the manufacturer (and six others) on the grounds that the labels were misleading because they implied that the absence of genetically engineered ingredients distinguished the product from competing brands, when actually, no genetically engineered wheat is present in any food. The manufacturer removed the label.

THIRD-PARTY LABELING SERVICES CAN IMPROVE MARKET EFFICIENCY

Third-party labeling services—services offered by an entity other than the buyer or seller—can increase a label's value by increasing its reliability and credibility. These services improve market efficiency by reducing uncertainty for producers and search and information costs for consumers. By increasing the value of information, third-party services can also boost the amount of information that producers provide to consumers through product labels. The four primary third-party labeling services are standard setting, verification, certification, and enforcement. A single entity could provide just one service or any combination of all four services.

- Through standard setting, third-party authentication helps ensure consumers that a firm's quality standards are meaningful for differentiation and are not simply empty marketing ploys. For example, "green," "sustainable," or "fair trade" could mean almost anything. Successful third-party standards establish a common terminology for goods possessing the same quality characteristics.
- Verification services can take the form of either testing (such as testing that pathogen contamination or other safety problems are under control) or process verification (such as inspecting production facilities and bookkeeping records to verify that firms have adhered to safety and quality standards and followed specified production practices) or segregation and traceability monitoring to verify the existence of process attributes, such as organic, fair trade, dolphin-safe, and sustainable. These services help producers strengthen their labeling claims by providing an objective measure of product attributes.
- Third-party certification provides evidence that testing and/or process verification has been completed and that the information supplied by firms or third-party verifiers is correct. Third-party certification provides an objective evaluation of the product's quality attributes and helps firms establish credible market claims. Through accreditation, third-party certification can also establish the credentials of other third-party services, including other third-party certifiers. For example, USDA accredits third-party certifiers for the National Organic Program.

- Third-party enforcement provides further assurances that quality claims are valid. Private third-party enforcement includes watchdog services and de-certification. Watchdog-type enforcement relies on negative publicity to discourage fraud. Firms with valuable reputations will be most susceptible to this type of enforcement. De-certification provides a clear indication that a product has failed to comply with quality standards. De-certification by government entities could carry the added penalty of prohibiting marketing of the product. Legal requisites concerning advertising and fraud provide the ultimate enforcement, even for voluntary claims.

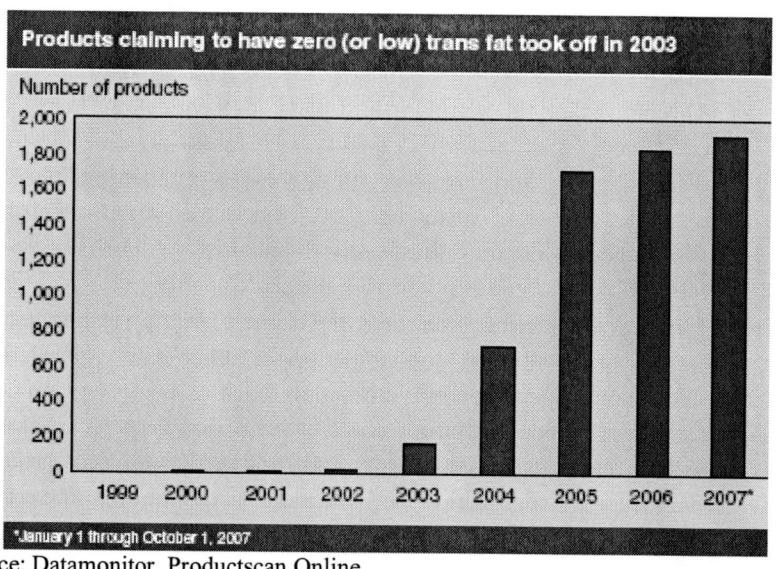

Source: Datamonitor, Productscan Online.

MANDATORY LABELING HAS TARGETED INFORMATION GAPS AND SOCIAL OBJECTIVES

U.S. Government intervention in labeling began in 1906 with the Federal Pure Food and Drugs Act and the Federal Meat Inspection Act, which authorized Federal regulation of the safety and quality of food and prohibited sales of misbranded or adulterated foods. Lawmakers' primary objective in passing the acts' labeling regulations was to enhance fair competition by cracking down on deceptive marketing practices.

Enhancing fair competition and market efficiency has remained a primary motivation behind food labeling regulation for the past 100 years. Regulations ranging from the 1966 Fair Packaging and Labeling Act (requiring all consumer products in interstate commerce to contain accurate information to facilitate value comparisons) to the Organic Foods Production Act 1990 have sought to create a level playing field for producers by providing consumers with accurate information for comparing products and making choices. These regulations seek to increase informed consumption, not to alter consumption behavior. USDA's National Organic Program (the result of the Organic Foods Production Act) is designed to improve the comparability of organic labeling claims, not persuade more consumers to choose organic products.

Recently, government intervention in labeling has begun to target environmental or other spillovers associated with food production and consumption. Individual food consumption decisions can have social welfare consequences, including effects on the environment, health and productivity, labor conditions, and farm and industry structure. For example, consumers who eat tuna caught with encircling nets may inadvertently endanger dolphins.

Economists describe these kinds of situations, in which the action of one economic agent affects the well-being or production possibilities of another in a way that is not reflected in market prices, as externalities.

When private consumption decisions result in externalities, social welfare may be maximized by a labeling choice that differs from one generated by private firms.

In the tuna example, the potential benefits of providing information on labels include fewer dolphin deaths. For society as a whole, these potential benefits may outweigh the increase in profits that compose a private firm's labeling benefits. As a result, the social benefits of labeling may outweigh the social costs even though the private benefits do not outweigh private costs. The opposite could also be true. For example, the increased consumption of red wine resulting from labeling red wine with the information that moderate consumption may lower the risk of heart disease could result in higher costs from more birth defects, car accidents, and alcohol-related health costs. These social costs may outweigh the benefits of reduced Heart disease.

On the other hand, the firm's net benefits may be positive: the costs of redesigning labels could be lower than the benefits of increased sales triggered by the health claim.

In externality cases where private firms do not supply relevant information, the government may decide to intervene in labeling decisions to try to maximize net social benefits. Government-mandated labeling can be a useful tool for achieving social objectives because of the potential power of information to influence consumption decisions. However, economic theory suggests that labels may be a poor means of addressing problems of externalities and advancing social objectives, such as protecting consumer health or the environment.

Even if some consumers alter their behavior to account for externality costs, others do not, which means that the objective will probably not be met. For example, while some may purchase only free-range chickens, their goal of ending chicken cooping will not be achieved as long as most consumers continue to buy chickens raised in coops.

Economic theory identifies a number of policy tools that may be more suited to redressing externalities than information remedies. Bans, quotas, production regulations or standards, and Pigouvian taxes (which impose the externality cost of an activity on its producer) may be more successful than mandatory labels in adjusting consumption and production to better match socially optimum levels.

Empirical studies have found mixed results on the efficacy of labels in educating consumers and changing consumption behavior. These studies highlight the observation that consumers often make hasty food choices in grocery stores and usually do not scrutinize food labels.

Researchers from Purdue University and the Ecole Nationale Superieure de Genie Industriel in France found that most participants in a marketing experiment did not notice the "GMO" (genetically modified organism) label on a food product until the label had been projected in large letters on a big screen.

Research also shows that a large number of warnings or a list of detailed product information may cause many consumers to disregard the label completely. And, even if consumers do consider each piece of information on a label, they may find it difficult to rank the information according to importance.

For example, out of 10 warnings on a label, consumers may have difficulty picking out the most important. As a result, consumers may underreact to important information or overreact to less important information.

LABELS MAY INFLUENCE PRODUCERS MORE THAN CONSUMERS

The primary impact of mandatory labeling regulations may stem from their effect on product reformulation and innovation, not on consumers' food choices.

Changes in labeling regulations can open up areas of competition by allowing producers to compete on a new set of attributes, like health claims. To compete in these new areas, manufacturers may introduce new or reformulated products.

Economists at the Federal Trade Commission found that regulation allowing health claims on cereal boxes resulted in significant product innovation and a plethora of cereals claiming to help reduce the risk of cancer. New labeling requirements can also spur product introductions or reformulations.

Firms that are forced to disclose the negative characteristics of their products may choose to reformulate rather than risk losing sales from disclosure.

Manufacturers' reactions to labeling policy could be quite swift. In an effort to be the first to label—and capture firstmover profits—manufacturers may reformulate before consumer demand kicks in.

FDA researchers found that leading up to mandatory trans fat labeling, most consumers did not know whether trans fats were good or bad. Nevertheless, in anticipation of mandatory labeling, manufacturers quickly jumped on the "no trans fat" bandwagon. From January 2005 through the first 9 months of 2007, manufacturers introduced 5,459 products with labeling touting low or zero trans fat content.

Manufacturers may label and reformulate even though most consumers are not particularly interested in the new attribute. Sometimes a small niche group of consumers is enough to warrant the expense of reformulation and product innovation, particularly when the new ingredient or attribute does not affect taste or price and therefore does not alienate core groups of consumers. The more attributes manufacturers can stack in their products—eco-friendly, low-sugar, fairtrade, high-fiber—the more niche consumers they may be able to attract.

As a result of product reformulation, labeling regulation can affect consumer food choices more than would have been accomplished simply via consumers' reactions to labels. Even consumers who remain indifferent to or unaware of a new attribute may consume more of it if their usual food choices have been reformulated.

For example, some consumers of popular snack foods may not know that their favorite nibbles are now made without trans fats. They are reaping the benefits of a potentially more healthful diet without changing their food choices. However, if the price of their favorite snack rises because of reformulation, consumers who do not want the new attribute are made worse off.

The benefits and costs of labeling regulation could be far reaching when manufacturers respond by reformulating. A shift to "zero trans fat" has triggered changes all along the processed food chain, including investments in new processing technologies and the development of soy and canola crop varieties with different oil characteristics. Other reformulations could have ramifications for the environment, animal welfare, and consumers' health and budgets.

These cases stand in stark contrast to those in which labels go unread and unnoticed.

They also underscore the potential of labeling policy that works with industry incentives to affect the content and quality of American diets.

INDEX

A

access, 10, 61
accounting, 20, 26, 27, 61
accreditation, 67
acid, 31
additives, 60
adults, 23, 30
advertisements, 8, 14, 17
advocacy, 66
age, 23, 24, 31, 61
age-related diseases, 31
aging population, 40
aging process, 31
allergic reaction, 29
allergy, 61
anaphylaxis, 29
animal welfare, 72
antioxidant, 28, 30, 31
antioxidants, vii, 2, 3, 28, 29, 31, 39, 52
apples, 64
arthritis, 31
assessment, 65
attitudes, 11
authentication, 67
authority, 8
autism, 30
awareness, 3, 31

B

baby boomers, 31
background information, 18
benefits, 6, 11, 13, 15, 18, 21, 25, 30, 31, 37, 40, 61, 64, 69, 70, 72
beverages, 5, 17, 27, 28, 39, 51
bones, 10
brand image, 26
buyer, 67

C

calcium, 8, 10, 12, 19, 21, 29, 30, 52
caloric intake, 27
calorie, vii, 2, 4, 19, 20, 21, 22, 27, 28, 39, 43, 60, 61
campaigns, vii, 2, 3, 39
cancer, 31, 71
car accidents, 69
carbohydrate, 21, 26, 29, 52, 61
cardiovascular disease, 31
cardiovascular function, 31
carotene, 31
category a, vii, 2, 17, 27, 28
CBS, 24
Celiac Disease, 29, 45, 46, 47
certification, 65, 67, 68
challenges, 30
chemicals, 60

Chicago, 29, 47
chicken, 70
childhood, 25
children, viii, 11, 23, 25, 61, 63
cholesterol, vii, 2, 3, 8, 10, 18, 19, 20, 21, 29, 52, 60
chronic diseases, 31
classification, 14
CNN, 24
coconut oil, 60
coffee, viii, 37, 63
cognitive function, 31
commerce, 69
common symptoms, 61
community, 31
competition, 3, 10, 16, 17, 37, 64, 65, 69, 71
competitive advantage, 7
competitive process, 3, 66
competitors, 6
complement, 4
compliance, 8
consensus, 31
consulting, 30
consumer choice, 6
consumer education, 65
consumer purchases, vii, 2, 4, 5
consumers, viii, 3, 4, 5, 7, 11, 12, 13, 18, 19, 21, 22, 25, 26, 27, 28, 30, 31, 37, 39, 40, 61, 63, 64, 65, 66, 67, 69, 70, 71, 72
consumption, viii, 4, 11, 12, 17, 22, 25, 26, 27, 31, 39, 63, 66, 69, 70
contamination, 67
cooking, 17
cost, 21, 25, 26, 70
credentials, 68
crop, 72
customers, 61

D

data collection, 14
database, 4, 12, 14, 15, 16, 18, 19, 20, 22, 24, 26, 27, 29, 34, 35, 37, 51, 52, 56, 59, 61
deaths, 69

defects, 69
deficit, 30
Department of Agriculture, 1
Department of Health and Human Services, 8, 18, 31, 37, 48, 49, 60, 61
depression, 30, 31, 61
diabetes, 30, 31
diet, 4, 5, 10, 11, 12, 25, 28, 30, 31, 37, 40, 72
Dietary Guidelines, 12, 25, 27, 31, 39, 41, 48, 49
Dietary Guidelines for Americans, 12, 25, 27, 39, 41, 48, 49
disclosure, 3, 6, 10, 31, 66, 71
diseases, 31
disorder, 30
distribution, 6, 35, 36
DNA, 31
dressings, 20, 51, 53, 54, 55, 56, 57, 59

E

Economic Research Service, 1, 47, 48, 63
economic theory, 70
economics, viii, 64
editors, 14, 44
education, vii, 2, 12
egg, 65
encouragement, 61
enforcement, 8, 22, 66, 67, 68
environment, 17, 69, 70, 72
epidemic, 24, 39, 61
equilibrium, 22
ERS, 64
ethnicity, 61
evidence, 10, 31, 61, 67
externalities, viii, 63, 69, 70

F

family-run farms, viii, 63
farms, viii, 63
fat, vii, 2, 3, 4, 5, 8, 12, 17, 18, 21, 22, 27, 29, 35, 38, 52, 53, 54, 57, 58, 60, 66, 71, 72

fatty acids, 3, 8, 13, 31, 33, 39, 60
FDA, 7, 8, 10, 18, 31, 39, 45, 47, 49, 50, 60, 61, 65, 66, 71
fiber, vii, 2, 3, 4, 8, 12, 18, 20, 21, 22, 23, 25, 27, 28, 29, 30, 39, 52, 61, 71
financial, 7
financial reports, 7
fish, 17, 21, 50, 51, 53, 54, 55, 56, 57, 58, 59
flavor, 5, 30
flour, 30
food, vii, viii, 2, 3, 4, 6, 7, 8, 12, 14, 15, 16, 17, 19, 20, 22, 24, 25, 29, 30, 31, 33, 35, 36, 37, 38, 39, 40, 48, 51, 52, 58, 59, 60, 61, 63, 64, 65, 66, 67, 69, 70, 71, 72
Food and Drug Administration, 7, 8, 49, 65
food chain, 72
food industry, 25, 33, 61, 64
food production, viii, 63, 69
food products, vii, 2, 3, 6, 36, 37, 38, 39, 40, 65
food safety, 65
force, 26
Ford, 11, 41, 45
formation, 60
formula, 35
France, 70
fraud, 68
freezing, 13
fruits, 13, 17, 65

G

gluten, vii, 2, 3, 13, 28, 29, 30, 33, 39, 52, 53, 57, 61
government intervention, 69
governments, viii, 64, 65
growth, vii, 2, 3, 5, 22, 26, 27, 28, 31, 37, 39, 61
guidance, 8, 61
guidelines, 7, 25, 26, 27
guilt, 12

H

harmful effects, 31
health, vii, viii, 2, 3, 4, 6, 7, 8, 10, 11, 12, 14, 16, 17, 18, 19, 20, 21, 22, 24, 25, 28, 29, 30, 31, 35, 36, 37, 38, 39, 40, 50, 51, 52, 53, 57, 60, 61, 63, 64, 66, 69, 70, 71, 72
Health and Human Services, 31
health care, 40
health care costs, 40
health information, 11
health problems, 25, 28, 31
healthfulness, 11, 12, 33, 37
heart disease, 10, 26, 31, 69
high blood pressure, 8
history, 7
hives, 29
House, 65
human, 7, 31
human body, 31
human right(s), 7
hyperactivity, 30
hypertension, 8
hypothesis, 16, 22

I

image, 6
immune system, 61
incidence, 31
income, 61
industries, 5
industry, 19, 27, 69, 72
ingredients, viii, 4, 6, 11, 13, 14, 30, 31, 33, 60, 63, 66
international standards, 65
intervention, 68
investments, 72
investors, 7
IRI, 4, 6, 31
iron, 8, 30
issues, 17, 22, 30

K

kicks, 71

L

labeling, vii, viii, 2, 3, 4, 7, 8, 22, 24, 26, 33, 39, 61, 63, 64, 65, 66, 67, 68, 69, 70, 71, 72
lactose, 52
lead, vii, 2, 11, 12, 16, 28, 31, 37
legislation, 7
life expectancy, 31
light, 8
litigation, 6
lutein, 65

M

magazines, 8, 14, 60
malnutrition, 28
management, 46
manufacturing, 10, 13
market failure, viii, 64
market share, 5
marketing, 4, 12, 13, 25, 37, 39, 60, 66, 67, 68, 69, 70
marketing strategy, 39
marketplace, 66
mass, 14, 34, 36
meat, 8, 17, 21, 50, 51, 54, 60
media, 11, 24
messages, 4, 13, 39
Metabolic, 41
metabolism, 31
molecules, 31
monosodium glutamate, 29, 52
mortality, 31
motivation, 69
multiple sclerosis, 30

N

National Health and Nutrition Examination Survey, 25
natural food, 34
nausea, 29
net social benefit, 70
nonprofit organizations, 60
nutrient(s), vii, 2, 4, 5, 6, 7, 8, 10, 11, 12, 15, 16, 17, 18, 19, 20, 22, 25, 29, 31, 33, 36, 37, 38, 39, 40, 60, 65
nutrition, vii, 2, 3, 4, 8, 10, 11, 12, 16, 17, 18, 19, 20, 22, 23, 24, 29, 30, 31, 36, 37, 38, 39, 40, 50, 51, 52, 53, 57
Nutrition Facts, vii, 2, 3, 7, 11, 12, 18, 31, 37, 39, 42, 44, 45
Nutrition Labeling and Education Act of 1990 (NLEA), vii, 2, 7, 8
nutrition labels, 12
nutrition-related claims, vii, 2, 3, 4, 11, 12, 16, 18, 19, 20, 22, 24, 29, 38, 50, 52, 53, 57

O

Obama, 25
obesity, vii, 2, 3, 22, 23, 24, 25, 27, 39, 60
oil, 17, 33, 60, 72
olive oil, 60
omega-3, vii, 2, 3, 8, 13, 28, 29, 30, 31, 39, 52, 65
Organic Foods Production Act, 69
organism, 70
osteoporosis, 28, 30
outreach, 64
overweight, 12
oxidation, 31
oxygen, 31

P

palm oil, 33
parents, 11
participants, 70

pasta, 21, 55
petroleum, 14
playing, 69
policy, 8, 36, 70, 71, 72
polyunsaturated fat, 65
polyunsaturated fatty acids, 65
population, 11
potential benefits, 69
poultry, 8, 17, 21, 50, 51, 53, 54, 55, 56, 57, 58, 59, 65
President, 5, 50
private benefits, 69
private costs, 69
private firms, 69, 70
probability, 64
producers, 11, 15, 21, 24, 67, 69, 71
product attributes, 67
product life cycle, 5
proliferation, 3
proposed regulations, 7
protection, 13
public awareness, 12
public health, 34
public interest, 6
pulp, 13

Q

quality control, 14
quality standards, 14, 67, 68
quotas, 70

R

radio, 37
reactions, 71
recognition, 26
recommendations, 5, 24, 25, 31, 61
red wine, 69
redistribution, 17
Reform, 47
regulations, viii, 2, 3, 4, 6, 7, 8, 10, 16, 17, 31, 33, 39, 60, 69, 70, 71
reliability, 7, 67
reputation, 7, 65

requirements, viii, 8, 10, 18, 26, 31, 37, 64, 71
researchers, 11, 71
resources, 11, 14, 31
retail, 14
rheumatoid arthritis, 30
risk(s), 8, 10, 11, 12, 26, 31, 69, 71
risk factors, 31
risk perception, 12
rules, vii, 2, 3, 7, 8, 17, 31, 39

S

safety, 67, 69
saturated fat, 8, 10, 12, 33, 37, 52, 60
science, 60
segregation, 67
sensitivity, 61
services, 26, 65, 67, 68
small businesses, 37
social benefits, 69
social costs, 69
social welfare, 69
society, 69
sodium, 4, 5, 7, 8, 12, 18, 19, 20, 21, 29, 33, 37, 52, 60, 66
spillovers, viii, 63, 69
states, 8
statistics, 25
stomach, 61
stress, 31
stroke, 31
structure, 8, 10, 69
substitutes, 21, 33, 51
success rate, 6
suppliers, 61
sustainability, 7
sweeteners, 27, 29, 52

T

target, 14, 69
Task Force, 5, 50
taxes, 70
technologies, 6, 31, 72

technology, 13
testing, 67
texture, 30
tracks, vii, 2, 4, 35
trade, 14, 34, 60, 67
training, 14
trans fats, vii, 2, 3, 6, 29, 31, 33, 34, 39, 52, 61, 71, 72
trustworthiness, 65

U

U.S. Department of Agriculture, 17, 47, 48, 49, 63
UK, 50
United, 1, 31, 41, 43, 44, 46, 47, 60
United States, 1, 31, 41, 43, 44, 46, 47
USA, 43, 47
USDA, 8, 41, 65, 68, 69

V

variations, 38
varieties, 72

vegetables, 17, 51, 54, 55, 57, 58, 59, 65
vitamin A, 8, 12
vitamin C, 8, 12, 31
Vitamin C, 41
vitamin E, 31, 65
vitamins, 18, 19, 22, 25, 28, 29, 30, 39, 52

W

Washington, 43, 44, 45, 47, 48, 49, 64
water, 51
web, 35, 36, 61
websites, 7, 8, 14, 35
weight control, 25
weight gain, 60
weight loss, 30
weight management, 30
welfare, viii, 64
well-being, 69
White House, 5, 50
wood, 13
World Health Organization, 22, 24
worldwide, 65